Bedside Matters

Bedside Matters

A Journey through
Doctor–Patient Communication

Peter Tate
Retired General Practitioner
Dorset, UK

With editorial contributions from
Francesca Frame
General Practitioner
Cambridgeshire, UK

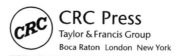

CRC Press
Taylor & Francis Group
Boca Raton London New York

CRC Press is an imprint of the
Taylor & Francis Group, an **informa** business

First edition published 2021
by CRC Press
6000 Broken Sound Parkway NW, Suite 300, Boca Raton, FL 33487-2742

and by CRC Press
2 Park Square, Milton Park, Abingdon, Oxon, OX14 4RN

Library of Congress Cataloging-in-Publication Data
Names: Tate, Peter, 1946- author. | Frame, Francesca, editor.
Title: Bedside matters : a journey through doctor–patient communication / author, Peter Tate ; with editorial contributions from, Francesca Frame.
Description: First edition. | Boca Raton : CRC Press, 2021. | Includes bibliographical references and index.
Identifiers: LCCN 2020021225 | ISBN 9780367467845 (paperback) | ISBN 9780367467852 (hardback) | ISBN 9781003031055 (ebook)
Subjects: MESH: Physician-Patient Relations
Classification: LCC R727.3 | NLM W 62 | DDC 610.69/6--dc23
LC record available at https://lccn.loc.gov/2020021225

ISBN: 9780367467852 (hbk)
ISBN: 9780367467845 (pbk)
ISBN: 9781003031055 (ebk)

Typeset in Minion Pro
by Nova Techset Private Limited, Bengaluru & Chennai, India

Contents

Introduction

It took some time to come up with the title for *Bedside Matters*, and in the end friends on Facebook helped; an unknown concept when I qualified in 1968. The sad truth is that doctors these days rarely sit by their patient's own bedside, but we are still judged on our bedside manner. I learned the hard way that what mattered to my patients had to matter to me, or I would remain a second-class physician. I have been retired now for 20 years, but the time felt right to look back over my medical career and reflect on the paths I took, the patients I met and the progress I tried to achieve in exploring and promoting patient-centred care.

Now of course, the world has been reminded what medicine is really about. I wrote this introduction at the end of March 2020, while everyone was reordering their priorities, reconsidering what really matters and learning to live with a frightening amount of uncertainty. Coping with uncertainty is the hardest subject young doctors must learn to deal with, and sharing that uncertainty is not usually welcomed by anxious patients. However, delivering a close approximation of the truth in a digestible form is the gold standard for any doctor. I learned this the hard way during my career; now all of us are having a harsh lesson about the realities of the inherent fragility of life imposed on us. Our lauded, but creaking, centralised health system is bureaucratically top-heavy, but if we are to learn only one thing from this crisis it must be to listen to people. In our search for excellence over mediocrity we have never needed focused, patient-centred care more. We need more trust and less paternalism, and doctors must start really listening to their patients and find the time to do so.

Personal and family experience of ill health focused my thoughts early in my career and helped me turn to the behavioural sciences. My trainer John Horder in particular sowed some early seeds, and I am forever indebted to David Pendleton, a then young social psychologist, who allowed me to join him and others on the quest for a better way of consulting. The Royal College of General Practitioners, especially the Panel of Examiners, became an integral part of my life. Working with friends such as Theo Schofield, Peter Havelock, Roger Neighbour, Tony Reed, David Haslam and John Foulkes, we tried to improve the understanding of the doctor–patient interface. The path has often been and remains bumpy, but it is a fascinating, never-ending journey that I have been so privileged to at least take a small part in.

What follows is a collection of essays covering at least half a century of trying to understand and improve communication between doctors and patients. It is not inclusive; by nature the essays are idiosyncratic, extremely personal and, of course, biased. The remembrances are as accurate as my fallible memory will allow, and everything I have written I believe to be true. Hoarding useless objects is a part of my character that infuriates my wife, but I kept diaries, magazine articles and newspaper cuttings over the years for the proverbial rainy day, and so when I felt the need to reminisce, there was all this material. The emotions locked in these dusty scraps shook me; pride, joy, despair, shame and embarrassment, all so powerful and so salutary. My wife, Judy, has sometimes found me typing away with tears falling unnoticed and unable to give her a coherent reason as to why; I suppose what follows is the best explanation I can do.

Some of the recollections are specialised and academic, but with the help of Francesca Frame, my co-author and editor, we have tried to separate out the driest bits into addenda for those who are really interested, while leaving the body of the text just about readable.

This book is intended for health professionals with an interest in the study of doctor–patient communication and not for a general prurient audience, but I have anonymised patient details as much as possible, while retaining as much truth as necessary to illustrate the point. I use these stories to demonstrate that clinical experiences, both professional and personal, are fundamental to our perception of what is important and what matters most in medicine.

Peter Tate
Poundbury, Dorchester
March 2020

1

Beginnings

I suspect we have always lived in troubled times. My life has its fair share of ups and downs and like most humans my optimism usually, but not always, trumps the pessimism. I can now look back with a reasonable depth of perspective, having achieved a feat that has looked unlikely most of my life; that of sailing past the three-score-and-ten limit.

My father, Ivan, was a single-handed general practitioner (GP) and, with only my mother as help, consulted from a damp basement surgery in Beach Road, South Shields. He had qualified aged 21 in 1937 from Durham, though his medical training, like mine, was in Newcastle. He had not wanted to be a doctor, he wished to be an Egyptologist, but his father and mother vetoed that. My grandfather, Robert Tate, was headmaster of St. Hilda's School, South Shields, and my grandmother Sally (née Scarfe) had been headmistress of Baring Street School, also in South Shields. They were loving, deeply Christian, Masonic and formidable. Dad, like me, was an only child. He went to South Shields Grammar School and proved bright. As a child I would come home from school to find him sitting on the stairs reading Wallis Budge's *Book of the Dead* and folding out long screeds of musty-smelling hieroglyphics. Mum thought him unhinged.

Four years after qualifying my father took his MD by examination early in the Second World War; he passed but told me of the most difficult question he was asked, 'What do you know about the aetiology of Crohn's disease?' He claimed he wrote 'I know very little about Crohn's disease at all'. I mention this because if asked the same question today, more than 70 years later, my answer would be very similar to my father's. Medicine is advancing but there are still vast swathes that we do not fully understand; something society struggles to accept.

Soon after qualification Dad ran away to sea, joining the SS Theseus, a Blue Funnel cargo and passenger ship, a part of Alfred Holt's navy, that sailed from Liverpool in late 1938. She was an old, slow ship, launched from Belfast in 1908 and had survived a fight with the Germans in the First World War; she would survive others in the new war. The homeward bound cargo was copra (dried coconut kernels) and he lived the rest of his life with a total hatred of *Necrobia rufipes*, the Copra Beetle. It infested the whole ship and if you were thirsty at night your water glass usually contained several of them mixed with the odd cockroach. Medically, Dad did very little, but he did manage to contract *Plasmodium vivax*, the lesser and commoner form of malaria, claiming that the necessary ingestion of quinine-laced tonic water fueled his love of gin. The SS Theseus was in Marseilles when the Second World War broke out and father, without the appropriate dockside pass, managed to rejoin the ship by waving his tailor's bill authoritatively. Or at least that is the tale he told. Later, SS Theseus was up near Narvik, Norway and came under fire from no less than the German battle cruiser Scharnhorst; she didn't sink, but Dad claimed he put on his dinner jacket to go out in style.

After the war, my father joined up with Dr Herbert Crisp as the junior partner in a general practice in South Shields. Herbert had been the family doctor forever; he had even delivered my father in 1917. In 1946, the year I was born, general practice was very different from now in so many ways. Perhaps the most important difference was the lack of clear split between hospital doctors and GPs. Herbert was a consulting physician to the Ingham Infirmary; he admitted patients there and looked after them in the hospital. He was a surgeon if the need arose, and routinely took out tonsils at home. He would do his own anaesthesia too, a terrifying thought to modern doctors. He was also required to be an obstetrician, but his obstetrics was much more brutal and unforgiving than now. This was still an era when society accepted that childbearing was risky and that both mothers and children could, and not infrequently did, die. I still have a collection of his obstetric implements; tubes for puncturing heads to suck out brains to allow delivery and at least save the mother, a gadget to decapitate stuck babies, as well as the normal array of long, short and curved forceps. Herbert taught my father to take a bucket with him when delivering a baby. The bucket was for drowning deformed babies. You may feel this description is unnecessarily frank, but medicine has always been brutal; there is an underlying rawness related to the struggles between life and death that our society does its best to screen us from.

In 1948 Aneurin Bevan imposed the National Health Service (NHS) on an unwilling profession. Dad hated the NHS; he thought it a patronising, intrinsically second-class system, fundamentally Stalinist and designed to produce mediocrity, not excellence. He also despised the British Medical Association (BMA) for letting him down and felt betrayed for the rest of his career. Dad had to take a decision he did not want to make, to stay in hospital or to make his life as a GP. Bevan had left no halfway house. Herbert was getting old and needed him, so in the end there was no choice.

In order to make the new health service work Bevan needed to get the powerful doctors on his side. He decided to pay those doctors remaining in hospital generously, the newly created 'Consultants'. 'I will stuff their mouths with gold', he is reputed to have said. He also encouraged contracts to allow Consultants to do private work to subsidise their earnings. The remaining GPs got none of this, and their pay dropped dramatically as traditional income sources were subsumed by the hospitals. GPs became second-class citizens overnight; the day of the generalist was gone.

In 1952 Lord Moran, Churchill's physician, compounded the gloom for GPs by describing them as those that had fallen off of the hospital ladder. The fact that this was unadulterated piffle has not stopped these beliefs being carried on to the present day, by hospital doctors and some of the public. Is it easier to know a lot about a little, or a little about a lot? It is a circular, unhelpful argument, but it is unarguable that the loss of generalists in hospitals has not helped patients.

What I did learn from my childhood was how pervasive medicine is. In my early teens I asked my mother why she had never taken me to the beach like other mothers. She looked amazed at my ignorance and lack of perspicacity. 'Why? Because we were always on duty!' No mobile phones then, no deputising service, simply genuine 24-hour commitment. The family and the job were inseparable. My mother's favourite story from this time was one night when father came in from his second night visit and the phone rang again; she answered and Dad, recognising the voice as an overanxious regular, was gesticulating, almost silently, to say he was out. My mother did her best, but at last the frustrated patient said, 'Well if the doctor is not in can I speak to the man in bed with you!' Mum was a bank teller by training but spent her married life working as a receptionist, nurse, counsellor, secretary, manager, and dragon at the door. Marrying a doctor is still not easy, but then it was a life sentence. It remained that way at least until the mid-1980s.

My first limited experience with illness and faulty communication came via my father. He became slower, felt indefinably below par and on occasions, embarrassingly, slurred his words. This was 1960, he was 43, a heavy smoker (always the red, flat-packed Du Maurier) and no mean gin drinker with a history of a severe depressive episode requiring inpatient admission and electroconvulsive therapy (ECT) a decade earlier. There is a cartoon of him at this time, drawn by the artist of the Shields Gazette.

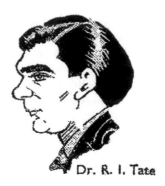

Dr. R. I. Tate

His very good friend was Henry Miller, then Dean of Newcastle Medical School, and one of the most admired neurologists in the country. They had been at Durham together and kept in touch. Henry was a bon viveur, a larger than life theatrical character, with immense charm and wit. Dad consulted him about his symptoms. Henry was not impressed and rang my mother without father's knowledge to say that dear Ivan was getting more hypochondriacal as the years went on and should cut down on the gin and fags. Mother was unimpressed, but Dad had a stab at cutting down and soldiered on.

Nearly three years went by and, by some fluke or misjudgment on Newcastle University's part, I started there on 2nd September 1963, my 17th birthday. I had been away at boarding school, but once back at home it was obvious that Dad was increasingly unwell but pig-headedly soldiering on; his friend had told him he was ok so he would get through it. We persuaded him to go back, Henry was unsure and sent him for a second opinion from his deputy and rapidly rising star John Walton. After a couple of tests and a brief admission the diagnosis of myasthenia gravis was made. I think Henry was mortified. I do know that in my entire time at university he never spoke to me once, claiming later that he did not know I was Ivan's son. He did you know.

In July 1968 Newcastle University let me loose, very young at only 21, with a head full of medical lore and a very limited concept of what being a doctor meant, despite my father being a battle-hardened GP. Consulting in the modern sense had not been on the curriculum. I vaguely half-remembered a couple of quotes from Sir William Osler, Professor of Medicine at Oxford, who had remarked that '*the good physician treats the disease the great physician treats the patient who has the disease*' and '*listen to the patient – she is telling you the diagnosis*'. These sort of aphorisms had only just managed to impinge on my consciousness, but were floating in the 'not quite important' part of my cortex. What, after five years, had been hammered into my mid-brain was 'taking a history'.

The nature of the game was diagnosis, most commonly demonstrated by often theatrical professors with a flare and mystery reminiscent of the best magicians. As in a conjuring trick, the patient supplied a few choice words (the professor made the choice) and hey presto, a magical name was pronounced. The diagnosis and all that subsequently followed were cloaked in a mystical, paternalistic obfuscation. Prescriptions were still written in Latin and patients were not encouraged to explore the nature or the consequences of their illness too deeply.

There was a long tradition behind this behaviour, dating back to Hippocrates. His famous, but rather weird, oath makes no reference at all to a doctor's duty to converse with patients. In fact, in *Decorum*, Hippocrates admonishes doctors to '*perform their duties calmly and adroitly, concealing most things from the patient ... revealing nothing of the patient's future or present condition*'. Plato, in several of his writings, stated categorically that doctors had a right to tell lies for good and noble purposes. This Greek ethic was rooted in the best of motives; it was believed that without respect for medical authority there could be no cure. The idea of the patient participating in decision-making was seen as counterproductive. The main tenets of Greco-Roman medicine were that patients must honour doctors, for the latter received their authority from the gods, and therefore patients must have faith in their doctors and promise obedience.

In the eighteenth and nineteenth centuries a few isolated luminaries suggested educating and involving patients. John Gregory, Professor of Medicine at Edinburgh, was a notable example. Benjamin Rush, a famous American contemporary of Gregory, held similar views, but, like Gregory, favoured deception whenever enlightenment was not equal to the task. They were both essentially pragmatists, seeking the most effective doctor–patient relationship for therapeutic ends. But by the middle of the nineteenth century some patients were beginning to get a little restless. John Stuart Mill, the famous libertarian, put it quite succinctly in 1859, '*Over himself, his own body and mind, the individual is sovereign*'. However, even by 1968, this view had not made too much of a dent in the cast iron medical school curriculum.

For the first few years of my medical career I therefore gave communication little thought and, like my father, had some fun as a ship's doctor. I joined the large (for its time) P&O liner SS Orcades in July 1969, having queued at the Hallam Street HQ of the General Medical Council (GMC) that morning to get the appropriate certificate. My time at sea was a unique adventure and hugely educational both in medical terms and in life experience. There are too many stories to relate here but I have published a memoir of that time, called *SeaSickness*. I will, however, relate my encounter with one of the most horrible diseases that ever existed. It was during my second spell at sea, now promoted to Ship's Surgeon, still on the P&O liner SS Orcades, when we were in the Northern Territories.

Darwin in North Australia is a strange place, and in 1971 its charms were certainly limited. There was a feeling of isolation about this town. The most exciting shop was Woolworth's, and the sidewalks were still more reminiscent of Tombstone than a modern city. A year later a terrible typhoon did untold damage, but here on Christmas Eve 1971 a chain of events, much less dramatic but of more personal significance, was about to unfold. The ship had been delayed because of electrical trouble in the boiler room, and while 12 hours in Darwin is a long time, three days seemed like a lifetime. A sort of torpid languor had engulfed passengers and crew alike; just how many times can you stare at the range of insect repellents and rat poisons which seemed to be Woollies' main stock? Still, we cleared them out of fairy lights and artificial snow, but Christmassy it wasn't. A few of the crew dressed up in coats, scarves and gloves and went carol singing. They carried lanterns and sang about gathering winter fuel and being in the deep midwinter as the temperature hovered around 100°C in the shade. Mad dogs and Englishmen.

I awoke on that Christmas morning gloomily contemplating the prospect of another very long day, while partaking of a breakfast in bed of Benson and Hedges and very black coffee. The sticky inertia was suddenly broken by a sharp knock and the immediate presence of Martin Le Tocq, the Assistant Surgeon. He looked worried, despite his festive party hat. I offered him a cigarette, gratefully accepted, and he told me he had a patient in the Crew Surgery who was giving him some concern.

The patient was Goanese and was one of a batch of 20 or so crew that had been flown into Singapore some five days ago to relieve others due leave. His problem was spots and slight fever. The anxiety to Martin, whose medical school would have been proud of him, was the nature of the spots. They were on the young man's arms and chest, raised from the surface of the skin, with a central dimple, and in medical jargon 'umbilicated'.

All the internal red lights went on at once; we looked at each other, eyes full of a mixture of fear, perplexity and with a little frisson of longed-for excitement. We jointly articulated a sort of 'it can't be, can it?' And in no time at all we were both down in the Surgery poring over this increasingly perplexed and anxious young man's spots.

Martin was right, this was an unusual rash. The differential diagnosis was both mundane and terrifying. Chickenpox was favourite, followed by insect bites, or a sort of skin infection commonly called impetigo, but, and it was a very big but, the spots themselves matched the classical textbook description of smallpox. Was there smallpox where he came from? Goa, now an international package holiday centre, was then a small province of mainland India, notable for its Catholic religion, and its beautiful, but very poor, populace. P&O had a long-standing arrangement with Goanese employment organisations, and had been recruiting inexpensive male crew for several decades. Their religion and their temperament made them eminently suitable for services on big white liners, as waiters, cabin servants and cooks. They were, however, living in third world conditions at home, and several diseases, now extinct in more advanced countries, were still endemic in their own. The $64,000-dollar question; was smallpox one of these diseases?

It was still very early in the morning, about 7 am, and at last the ship was fixed and just setting out on its way to a stop at Hayman Island, a top tourist spot on the Great Barrier Reef. This was a good two days' sailing away. Now serious infectious disease anywhere is a terror, but on a passenger liner it is a disaster of Hollywood proportions, something that our world has recently been oh so brutally reminded of. Smallpox is one of the most infectious diseases we know of, much more so than COVID-19, and also has a truly frightening mortality, varying from nearly 100% to, at best, 20%–30%, depending on the strain of the virus and the susceptibility of the community it struck. In recent times, we have become accustomed to think of smallpox as a weapon of terrorism, since the disease itself was wiped out by the World Health Organisation's (WHO) vaccination programme in the 1980s. Even at the time of which I write, it was rare and confined to poor populations in hot countries. Doctors trained as we were had no actual experience of the illness, our knowledge was all theoretical and historical. However, there were still doctors who did have experience and here we were lucky. As a senior officer, I had my own table in the restaurant with eight allotted passengers, one of whom was a retired colonial medical officer, last stationed in Burma and now on his way home to England for the last time. I rang him and asked if he would mind coming to the surgery PDQ. He came without demur, the old medical antennae sensing a crisis and a chance to be useful. We showed him the young Goanese patient, Dominico, without priming him to our own fears. He was thorough and professional. We went into my office and he shook his head gravely. 'That's Variola (the Latin name for smallpox), or I'm a Dutchman. Probably Variola minor; a slightly attenuated version but still nasty and can sometimes revert back to the real McCoy'. He looked at us pityingly. 'Heck I am glad I am not in your shoes; and it's Christmas too'.

Martin and I suffered a mutual sinking feeling coupled with a sudden awareness of the deep trouble we, and everyone else on the ship, was now in. First things first, Dominico needed isolating. We were lucky in that respect; the ship's hospital was situated over the propeller and there was a small self-contained room designed for just this purpose, known as the Brig. It also doubled as a cell should the need for restraint arise in aggressive crew or passenger.

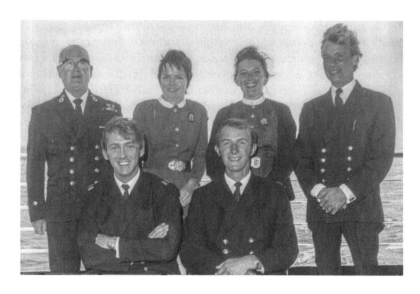

Medical Department SS Orcades, 1971.

Our attempts at doctor–patient communication were ineffective; Dominico became distressed, his English was poor, but it was clear that he disagreed with our diagnosis and he had to be strong-armed into the Brig. Of greater priority was telling the Captain what we were facing. This was my job and the prospect was not an attractive one. This was not because the Captain was an ogre, but he was hardly going to be a happy chappy when faced with a potentially lethal epidemic with 1,500 passengers off the Australian Coast. The Aussies were already renowned for being the fussiest nation on Earth when it came to health matters on ships, so they were not going to take kindly to this news, and neither was the Captain.

I said I was sorry to bother him at this hour; he told me to get on with it. I suggested he poured himself a gin; he said he never drank at this time of day and no news could be that bad. I said we had a case of smallpox on board and he asked if I would like a gin too. The Captain stared at me, asked how sure I was, and I told him of our experienced third opinion. We could be wrong, but the odds and the seriousness were such that we had to treat the risk as real. He gulped the large gin down in one and summoned the Staff Captain, Chief Officer and Purser. This was the gloomiest senior officer call I ever attended. Anger at the sheer unfairness of it all, and underneath a faint whiff of fear. This disease killed people; it could, given half a chance, kill lots of people, and senior ship's officers were not immune. I was asked for my recommendations. It sounds awful but I was starting to enjoy this situation in a vicarious sort of way. Here I was, 25 and Senior Surgeon, giving my advice to very experienced men much older than I. It was a big change from being a houseman, where I was used to being only one up from the hospital cat, and that was only when there were no mice around.

I said we needed to vaccinate everyone on board who could not produce a valid international certificate and inspect everyone on the ship every 24 hours for signs of the illness. The new arrivals from Goa should be quarantined and they should be inspected 12-hourly. We had enough vaccine on board for this purpose, having taken on a fresh batch in Singapore a few days earlier; it must have been a sixth sense. The Staff Captain wondered what and when should we tell the passengers, and the Purser wondered if we should shut the restaurant and feed everyone sandwiches. The Captain wondered to himself if this would be his last voyage.

We concocted a little note to be delivered to all passengers. It said that we had a case of smallpox on board, but it was mild and the patient had been isolated. Then we radioed the Darwin Port Health, who said we could not go back, and suggested talking to the authorities in Brisbane. Eventually the Captain spoke briefly, and I was handed the radio to talk to the Australian Chief Medical Officer (CMO). He was a cross-sounding man with no discernible sense of humour; not that the situation was funny. He insisted all on board should be inspected 24-hourly, but 12-hourly within 48 hours of landfall and yes, all on board without a valid certificate must be vaccinated, no excuses tolerated. He did give the impression that he was as certain as he could be that our diagnosis was wrong, and this was probably a storm in a teacup. We were to move out of Australian Territorial Waters and make our way to Brisbane for further instructions; the Great Barrier Reef stop was summarily cancelled.

This was going to be a logistic nightmare. The CMO had insisted only the ship's doctors could do the inspections but the nurses could help with the vaccinations. There were only two doctors, two nurses and Ron, the ex-naval dispenser who counted as a nurse as far as I was concerned. Fortunately, there was already an established inspection routine pre-docking in Australian ports. The Australian Port Health Authority ruled that any ship from non-Australian ports must undergo a full smallpox inspection prior to being allowed to dock, so there was an expectation of such from both the passengers and the crew. However, doing it for four days, and twice a day for the last two days, was going to severely test everyone's patience, and would finally put to the test the much-vaunted stamina of the two young doctors.

The Purser got all the crew together and told them the situation. Martin embellished a bit of medical detail to impress upon them the genuine seriousness of the situation. The Goanese took it especially badly, perceiving this event as a form of victimisation, a slur on their good name and hygiene, and all were convinced it was chickenpox misdiagnosed by sybaritic, wet behind the ears, just-out-of western medical school doctors.

To be honest, we were beset by doubt ourselves. In the 12 hours since diagnosis, Dominico was no worse physically, though emotionally he was far from chipper. Ron's jibes that he could have anything to eat that he wanted, as long it was flat and could be pushed under the door, was laboriously translated by the Chief Pantryman and lost any intrinsic humour, only producing loud sobs and wails of anguish from Dominico. We were now doing our best to barrier nurse him, but the green outfits which were full of holes due to the sheer age of the gowns, and rather full, dental-type face masks did nothing to make the poor soul feel cared for.

There was pressure from many passengers to have an explanatory meeting, so all were summoned to the main ballroom and the Staff Captain did his best. Suddenly it was my turn. It was disconcerting to suddenly feel the tension; my palms were sweating, and the heart was racing. The smile was too fixed, the denials of real danger a bit too strident, and I think the overall impression I created was of a recently decapitated chicken running in circles desperately trying to hold on to its head. We begged for understanding and patience and finally the mass meeting melted away. But the mood was not that of the Blitz, it was more like that just prior to the storming of the Bastille.

The Christmas buffet was cheering, extending as it did the full width of the recently cleared Ballroom. There were pig's heads with apples in their mouths, swans, snowmen and a huge white cockatoo all fashioned in marzipan, and an entire aquarium with brightly coloured fishes swimming in green aspic jelly. It did not make up for missing the Great Barrier Reef, but it was a start.

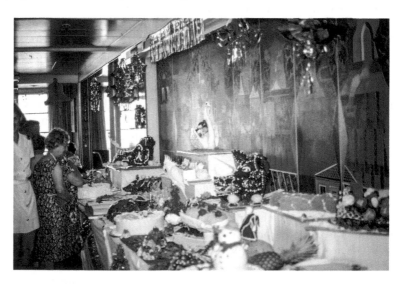

Christmas Buffet SS Orcades.

We also had our secret weapon; Magda. Magda was the formidable Dutch Woman Assistant Purser (WAP). She was stolid in form, thought and deed, but most significantly she also possessed a voice that would cowe tigers. The ship's public-address system was handed over to her to bark out the necessary instructions to the, as Magda saw it, inherently simple-minded, sheep-like passengers. She was magnificent; passengers simply obeyed orders barked out in this Teutonic accent which brooked absolutely no contradiction. With Magda in charge of orders, this puny disease did not have a chance.

Medically, we decided to combine the first inspection with the mass vaccination; we did the crew first to get our hand in, as it were. We decided to vaccinate all the Goanese crew whatever their smallpox certificate said. This was because, to a man, they were all notorious needle haters, and it was well known that most of the certificates were forged. Vaccinating was done by placing a drop of serum on the skin, scratching two parallel lines at right angles and rubbing the stuff in to the scratches with a needle. It was not a painful procedure, but the reaction of many would belie that fact. We brooked no excuses, however elaborate, and always handed the most recalcitrant over to Ron, who had an aura of immovability. The Purser also had a bright idea to put some backbone into the passengers; he played Verdi's Grand March from *Aida* at high volume from the ballroom speakers, and such stirring music did have a profound morale-lifting effect. To this day, if I hear it, I think of smallpox. We got to bed in the early hours and dreamt of spots, arms and pyramids. Orcades steamed up and round the North Australian Coast. The passengers went to bed early, with dampened, but not extinguished, Christmas spirits. Dominico cried himself into a fitful sleep, robotically fiddling with his Rosary, and a few more spots popped out just to keep the tension up.

The next morning Martin and I inspected the newly arrived Goanese with a fine toothcomb. We made them strip and peered at them all over; but luck was with us and no one else had spots. This inspection was much more thorough than we accorded the rest of the ship's complement. The accepted wisdom was that smallpox was a centrifugal illness and chickenpox a centripetal one. This meant the easy way to inspect for smallpox was to inspect forearms and face, as these were the likeliest places for the spots to first show themselves. Chickenpox mainly starts on the trunk. This however, like everything in medicine, is a guide, not a certainty. It also meant that we did not need to insist on passengers shuffling through disrobed, which was likely to start a riot, or at least uncontrollable giggling.

The mechanics of the passenger inspection were complex. The ballroom was assigned for the purpose. The two of us doctors were stationed towards one end on either side, and the passengers were divided into two rows that shuffled down towards us, rolling up sleeves as they came. Each doctor was assigned a WAP to check the passenger list and see that the names were properly ticked off; meanwhile male Assistant Pursers were assigned to general policing of the lines and seeking out recalcitrants. Magda continued to boom instructions out of the speakers, demanding passengers from various cabin numbers, and finally for the really tardy ones, naming names. 'Will Mrs Bloomstein from cabin three on C deck attend the smallpox inspection immediately'. The unspoken, but clear, message left hanging in the air was that Mrs Bloomstein would undoubtedly be shot if she continued to disobey orders.

For us inspectors, it was tedious work. Many passengers tried to eke out bits of information on how many fresh cases there were, and were palpably disbelieving when told still only one. The rumour machine already had us treating dozens in a secret location somewhere in the crew quarters. 'When are the proper doctors going to be flown in?' was a particularly irritating common refrain.

But there were compensations. In my case it was being assigned Sandra, the mysterious, beautiful, blonde WAP who had, so far this voyage, treated me with total scorn, but over these four days was eventually forced to talk to me out of sheer tedium. I was helped out by a young Australian mum who had named her daughter Galadriel; I remarked that she must be a Tolkien fan like me, and found out that Sandra was too. We talked of Tolkien and *Lord of the Rings*, swapping our favourite bits, discussing inconsistencies, and planning to make a film 30 years before they did. From there the conversation edged outwards. I learned about her best friends, her brother Chris and mother Dorothy, but nothing about her life except that she had once been a disc jockey in Corfu. By Brisbane I was hopelessly in love, and she was at least aware of my existence.

Dominico never became really ill, but by the time we neared Brisbane harbour he had an impressive array of spots in all stages of development. We were lucky in that no one else had developed the disease; our strategies had seemed to be effective. There was a cautious optimism about, but the Australian Port Health Authority did not share this feeling. They were taking no chances; we were not even allowed into the harbour, being told to anchor outside. We were also instructed to fly two yellow flags. Normally only one yellow flag was flown prior to being cleared by Port Health; two yellow flags signified we were a dangerous pariah.

Fortunately, it was a calm blue day, and as the passengers got word that the 'proper doctors' were coming, a large gathering appeared at the rails to watch for their arrival. After what seemed like an age, a disappointingly ordinary little launch pootled out to the ship. We were waiting at the main passenger door and the launch gangway was lowered. Three spacemen appeared, in full protection barrier suits with visors, white gloves and white Wellington boots. I couldn't understand anything the lead spaceman said to me as it was all muffled by the visor and deepest Australian, so I nodded, did a traditional thumbs up, and led them to the hospital anyway.

Dominico was beside himself with terror as this group entered the claustrophobic, dingy Brig. I tried to sooth him, but Ron just told him to shut up which seemed to work better. The last of the spacemen unpacked what seemed like a large piece of cling film and wrapped poor Dominico in it. He stuck a snorkel-like thing in his mouth and continued wrapping. A fourth spaceman appeared in the door, with light glowing from his visor and pushing a shiny hospital trolley. It really was surreal.

Dominico, trussed like a cooked chicken, was unceremoniously grabbed and dumped on the trolley and whisked away, his breathing tube poking through the wrapping. He looked like an insect chrysalis. We never saw him again. Nothing else happened for hours, and we remained bobbing somewhat nauseously at anchor, with the fleshpots of Brisbane tantalisingly visible. Eventually we received a radio communication from Port Health; we could lower one yellow flag and proceed to a berth, but no one was to disembark until further instruction and, almost as an afterthought, smallpox inspections were to continue 12-hourly till further notice. There was mutiny afoot; Brisbane was just too near for this forced incarceration to be tolerated long. Passengers besieged the ship's bureau, voices were raised, the Masters at Arms (ship's policemen) took up stations, and the Staff Captain and Purser fretted over strategies to defuse the tension, neither of them being able to think of anything very useful. The Captain got on the radio to P&O head office, known as 'The Company'. They must do something and soon, if strings need pulling well pull them now, or he would not be responsible for the consequences, which at that juncture looked like an imminent breakdown in civil order on the ship.

It was about this time that the Chief Pantryman, leader of the Goanese community, tapped me on the shoulder. Please come to the crew quarters, another crew member was sick and had spots! My legs momentarily went a bit funny and a strange fizzing feeling engulfed my head; my mouth really did go dry. I found Martin, summoned Ron, and off we went into the bowels of the ship. The smell of curry permeated the whole dingy warren that was the Goanese quarters. Our patient was cowering in the darkest part of a gloomy cabin; we could not see if he was wearing a shirt let alone if he had spots. Ron, used to this, had brought a huge torch with a beam like a searchlight; he shone it in the startled young man's eyes who promptly curled up firmly into the foetal position and could not be unravelled.

No amount of cajoling by an increasingly agitated Chief Pantryman made any difference. Ron threatened to hit him with the torch; that did it. He peeled off his shirt very reluctantly and revealed a panorama of spots, but my spirits soared; they were the wrong sort of spots. How do you recognise different sorts of spots you may ask? Dermatologists drum into medical students the basic types, and in the end, it is like recognising breeds of dog, an instantaneous recognition that would take a paragraph or two to describe. This chap had urticaria, colloquially often known as hives or an allergic rash. There are many causes of such a rash, the commonest being described medically as idiopathic or, to translate, not the faintest idea. But to my knowledge smallpox did not feature in the list of possible causes. Martin and I beamed at each other and basked briefly in mutually shared professional smugness. I said immediately to all present 'don't worry, this is not smallpox, this is urticaria, you can see he has classical target lesions, and look'. Here, I scraped the patient's skin with a handy spoon and a red wheal arose in the straight line that I had drawn. This was confirmation of the supercharged sensitivity of his skin. Just light pressure released enough histamine to produce a wheal and, as far as we were concerned, confirmed the diagnosis. The patient looked not unreasonably aggrieved, but was beginning to soften as he saw we were cheerful, and his worst fears were rapidly receding. Ron dispensed some antihistamine pills and the Chief Pantryman took us all to see the truly beautiful crib they had created. At least here on the ship, Christmas was celebrated with genuine piety, plus a little touch of entrepreneurial spirit, as it was quite clear we were expected to leave a donation for 'those at home'. In the circumstances we shelled out quite generously.

Panic over, we emerged back into the light in front of the Bureau (the ship's hotel reception) breathing more freely; our luck was still holding. Sandra's wasn't, she was in tears, as were two other WAPs, overcome by the sheer intolerance of the passengers. Only Magda was stoutly resisting the onslaught; the thought of Horatio holding the bridge came to mind. She firmly grasped the public-address system and yelled into it that all passengers must immediately return to their cabins to await further information on embarkation and that the Bureau was closing until further notice. Then with a powerful tug she unceremoniously pulled the shutters down.

At last the Port Health Authority came up with a ruling; all disembarking passengers should be inspected one last time and then allowed to leave, on the condition that they reported to Port Health every 24 hours for a further three days. All other passengers and crew were confined to the ship. We were to carry on inspections until Sydney, three days sailing away, and if there were still no more cases of smallpox, we would be declared infection-free. This was just enough to stop a riot, and the ship's entertainment staff were busy organising all manner of activities, including such cruising staples as frog racing, deck tennis contests and a passenger-based music hall. A spirit of the Blitz at last did materialise. Perversely, I now began to fret about the ending of the smallpox inspections. It was my main chance to monopolise the glamorous Sandra and press my suite; it had to be admitted that, though I was besotted, she was just mildly friendly and firmly resisted any more intrusive dating strategies.

This penultimate inspection at last had a view; Ball's Pyramid. This amazing, huge, sharp lump of basalt appears, arrowhead-like, in the Tasman Sea out of nowhere. It really is a pyramid and, to use that now overused expression, awesome. The Captain steered as close as he dared. On came the Grand March from *Aida* once again, and the passengers strode past our inspecting eyes with renewed vigour.

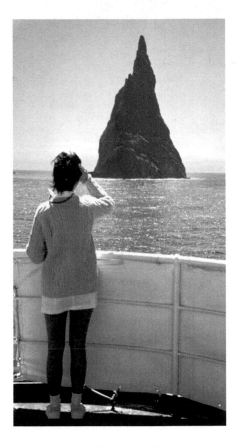

Ball's Pyramid.

At last it was all over. The ballroom deserted and the stunning vista of Sydney Harbour appeared through the gap known as the Heads. Sandra closed her passenger ledger and just stared; I was certain there was a tear in her eye. It gave me hope.

Though we made several enquiries, Brisbane Port Health Authority never confirmed our patient's illness as smallpox, but they never said it wasn't either. I remain convinced we saw the last case of smallpox on a passenger liner, and it did get me a wife.

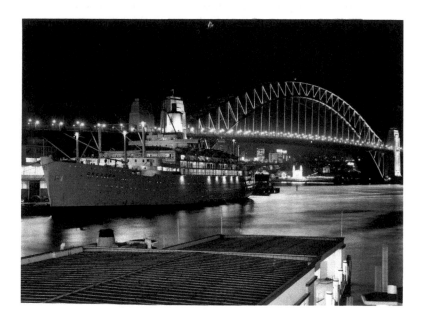

SS Orcades in Sydney Harbour 71.

REFERENCES

Mill J.S. 1982. *On Liberty.* New York: Penguin Classics.
Tate P. 2006. *Seasickness.* Lulu.com.

2

General Practice Beginnings

Being married meant I had to stop faffing about and make a choice. For the first time I began to think that I really wanted to be a GP, not least because I am left-handed, making my other choice, surgery, more difficult. Operating theatres then were very right-handed places, as were many instruments. I finally got off ship in late 1972 and moved in with my future wife in London. General practice training was not compulsory then and I toyed with going straight into practice, but a little inner voice told me I was nowhere near the finished article and that I needed more help. I applied for a traineeship in Kentish Town, and against the odds got it. To this day I can't get over how lucky I was.

The enthusiasm for general practice demonstrated by all in my training practice was infectious. This osmosed into my being over the year and has remained there ever since. Looking back, I can dissect out bits of specific enthusiasms that were demonstrated to me. My trainer, Mike Modell, was in the process of sitting the MRCP (Membership of the Royal College of Physicians) examination, having gone into general practice straight from house jobs, as you could in those days. The MRCP required an enormous amount of extra work. There was no obvious professional gain attached to this qualification for him at that time, just pride and proof that Lord Moran was wrong.

The practice had two trainers, giving different experiences and different perspectives. I quickly discovered that my other trainer was very special too. John Horder, thinker, painter, psychiatrist, polymath and flag carrier for the Royal College of General Practitioners (RCGP). My father was uncomfortable about the RCGP, like many of his colleagues, perceiving them as a southern-orientated group of self-important, regalia-obsessed losers who had made the wrong career choice, and whose self-aggrandizing behaviour was a Freudian manifestation of an implicit inferiority complex. He was wrong, but not totally. One of the founders, William Pickles, was a GP from Wensleydale, and had done some wonderfully rigorous and beautifully simple research into the spread of infectious disease in Yorkshire villages. His biography remains in print and is still well worth reading. It is a great testament to the generalist. Anecdotally, I shared a study with his grandson when I was a pupil at Giggleswick School in Yorkshire. At that school I had the luck to be inspired by a wonderful enthusiast for the English language and drama; he was Russell Harty who later became famous as a chat show host, and died far too young of an illness suspiciously like AIDS. In that same study another boy was inspired to take up acting, changed his name to Anthony Daniels, and achieved lasting worldwide fame as the very camp, intergalactic golden robot C-3PO.

Early on in my trainee year John Horder gave me a chapter in the newly published book *The Future General Practitioner* to read to form the basis of a tutorial. It was headed 'The Consultation' and began with this quotation from James Spence and Professor of Paediatrics at my own university:

> *The real work of a doctor is not an affair of health centres, or laboratories, or hospital beds. Techniques have their place in medicine, but they are not medicine. The essential unit of medical practice is the occasion when, in the intimacy of the consulting room or sick room, a person who is ill, or believes himself to be ill, seeks the advice of a doctor whom he trusts. This is a consultation, and all else in the practice of medicine derives from it.*
>
> *Spence 1938*

I had heard it before but given it no meaningful thought. The chapter described a theoretical approach to the consultation, and this defeated me. Exams at school were never that difficult and reading had been a joy; yet here was a set of words that made no sense to me at all. This was unfamiliar and terrifying. John, together with other luminaries ahead of their time, had written this stuff that I could not understand. Re-reading it now I could make some valid observations and suggest ways of lightening it up, but then, in 1973, it was just impenetrable. It was a good lesson. I was dimmer than I thought, but a seed had been sown.

The same trainer introduced me to the thoughts of Hungarian psychoanalyst Michael Balint and his book, *The Doctor, His Patient and the Illness*. John was a member of the original group, and Balint had died only a couple of years earlier. Although I never became a true disciple myself, the insights about the drug doctor and the role of emotions in consulting were revelatory and permanent. I had the cheek to write to my trainers as I came to the end of my year. There were three areas I delineated that had most improved my ability to help people. Firstly, listening properly to what patients say. Secondly, the skill of using time, both diagnostically and over a series of consultations to understand people better. And lastly, good note keeping, described as the root from which all else grows. I can hear my old partners' hollow laughter now.*

John Horder recognised that other sorts of general practice existed, and he sent me for a couple of days to a friend of his in Bourne End near High Wycombe on the Thames. I didn't know it then, but a young partner called Peter Havelock had just started, whose life was to intertwine with mine, but that is for later. The senior partner, Joe Bailey, was a genuinely larger than life character who drove a Rolls Royce and had a huge private practice. You must remember this was nearly 50 years ago. He dabbled in many therapies, but was particularly fond of manipulation. Being a huge man, six feet four inches and big with it, made his manipulative practice pretty impressive; patients flocked to him and his success rate was staggering. In his view the real element of the cure was the satisfying 'crack-crack' as the back was deftly twisted, and he confided in me that to obtain the best results, he always carried walnut shells in his pocket which he deftly crunched at the appropriate time to magnify the moment. Now that was healing.

* The other practice in the then new health centre was equally, but differently, progressive. Don Grant, then senior partner, was a dynamic and passionate socialist and the practice was modelled on egalitarian left-wing philosophy. Iona Heath was a trainee and then partner there a couple of years after my time. The politics were unfamiliar to me, as my father was probably a soft centrist urban Geordie Tory in a sort of Ken Clark style, and my mother, in her belief, was an unreconstructed right winger. What has always fascinated me about my mother's politics was her relationship with Joan. She was the family cleaner, looking after the house and the surgery. They both had long animated political discussions and, as far as I could tell, agreed on just about everything. Joan of course was a lifelong Labour voter, both of their opinions were often uncharitable in an Alan Bennett *Talking Heads* sort of way, but only divided by tribalism, which may explain why Brexit was such a mess for both main parties. My own training practice was of a gently left-leaning centrist persuasion. We had a branch surgery in Primrose Hill, and on the car journey over it was advisable to put the dropped cockney H's back, but I never have quite come to terms with the Hampstead/Islington hypocritical champagne socialism.

As a child we had had several riverboat holidays on the Thames which always seemed magical when compared to dear old South Shields, so when it came to choosing a practice, my wife and I chose the Thames Valley. Abingdon begins with A; it was the only job I applied for. My wife always regretted that it wasn't Henley. I went for interview in the pokey little surgery in Ock Street, and the cleaner whispered loudly to me that they were alright but the other surgery in the town was better. In fact, it was good place to spend 30 years.* I started in December 1973, when I joined Drs Adrian Semmence and Bob Pinches. Sandra and I bought a little old two-up two-down in Marcham, acquired a cat, and settled in very quickly. I took up cricket again.

Here was I, fresh out of general practice training, green as grass, an idealist, following a long tradition of young medics. I was going to sweep away the inefficiencies of my older colleagues. I would diagnose people, find all the diseases others had missed, I was going to make people better. Every surgery was an exciting challenge, every visit an adventure.

It was a Thursday in January 1974 that I was first called to visit Mabel Crump. The message gave the reason as 'legs'. Mabel lived in some council flats in the old centre of town only a few hundred yards from our Ock Street Surgery. The entrance was obscure, and it took several minutes to find it. It was the lady in the health food shop who put me out of my misery.

'You the doctor come for Mabel?'

I nodded self-consciously, carrying my overlarge new plastic doctor's bag and red stethoscope. She pointed to an alleyway.

'Down there, she's on the right. Take her vitamins every week I do. Funny old trout really'.

She looked at me properly with a squinting assessment.

'You're the new doctor? Gawd you don't look old enough to deliver newspapers'. She smiled, 'Good luck anyway'.

Mabel's door was ajar, and a smell emanated which I did not recognise then, but has become familiar to me over the years as that of human bodies past their best. The room was dark, curtains half drawn, and there by the

* The actual reason for choosing this practice was its forward thinkingness; it was a member of the Oxford Record Linkage system, a revolutionary pilot to combine GP and hospital records. Sadly, it did not work out too well and 50 years later we are not much further forward.

gas fire sat Mabel. I say sat, but this is a totally inadequate description. I don't think there is a word in the English language that truly describes her posture. She was slumped in the chair as if she had just fallen backwards into it; her vast blue legs were apart revealing a highly inadequate gusset. Sharon Stone she wasn't. She made an effort to focus on me, without any change in position.

'Who the fuck are you?'

I was unprepared for this greeting, stumbled over an object and became unbalanced because of my heavy, cumbersome bag, staggered dangerously towards her open crotch, stabilised myself just in time and mumbled unconvincingly.

'I am Dr Tate, the new doctor from the Ock Street Surgery'.

She looked at me with withering disbelief. I discovered an early truth then; people in their own houses have much more power than in my surgery. I was on her territory and she was boss. This was uncomfortable. There was a silence. A stale urine smell was emanating from the chair and empowered by the gas fire. My eyes started to water. What to say? I was not in control. She gestured with frighteningly deformed hands to what seemed to be her exposed nether regions.

'Me legs'. She said.

Silence fell again. I looked at her legs more closely. Below her knees on both legs were large ulcerated areas. The legs were massive. She was wearing slippers but no socks. Kneeling down to get a closer look, the carpet squelched and an unnerving sensation of creeping dampness embraced my knees. My senior partner's warning came to mind too late.

'Off to see Mabel are you, well you better learn the rules quickly. In a house like hers, and there are lots, there are only two rules but never forget them or I promise you, you will regret it. Never sit down and never kneel down. Rule two, never forget the first rule'.

I just had. While this unpleasant realisation was literally sinking in, my eyes, now more accustomed to the gloom could focus on the ulcers. They were huge, at least six inches across, covered in yellow foul-smelling pus, and no, surely not, there was movement. There were maggots. A wave of nausea hit me, I gagged and fought desperately against vomiting over the urine- and pus-enriched carpet.

That was the first visit, and all I saw then was a deformed, maggot-infested old crone who repulsed me. General practice was not going to be much fun if there were many Mabels. I was wrong, and she continued to teach me and over the months we became accustomed to each other. Friends would be the wrong word, but Mabel thought she needed me, and I became fascinated by her story.

When she was young, Mabel loved horses. Men were incidental, and her job at the Post Office only an interruption between the visits to the stable and the companionship of her beloved horse Elley. The day Elley died, part of Mabel died too. She never found a replacement, drifted into marriage with an outwardly dry and inwardly shrivelled professional photographer, had two children, both girls, who gave her no pleasure, and lived an arid, joyless English life. She was widowed at 60, both girls long gone abroad, as far from mother as they could get. Age had withered and rumpled Mabel; the bags under her eyes were spectacular, her jowls hung like a bloodhound and her chin folded like a well-used fan. The bottom eyelids began to fold outwards in this general collapse of the flesh, giving her a doleful doggy look that was both sad and a little macabre. By now she was heroically ugly, 16 stone with osteoarthritis of her hips and rapidly deforming hands, the knuckles swelling and the fingers falling sideways. When I met her, she had not set foot out of the door for five years. She was 72, a year younger than I am writing this recollection.

In fact, the district nurses heroically dressed and coped with her ulcers, the social services department set up an efficient care package. They got her up in the morning, Meals on Wheels ('Muck in a truck' according to Mabel) fed her, the nurse assistant bed-bathed her regularly and someone came to put her to bed. My role as her doctor was very peripheral, but to her, still crucial. In her mind I was what stood between her and the grim reaper. To me, I wasn't sure what to do, medical school hadn't really equipped me for this long-term, pastoral sort of care, but I had been taught to do things, and so I did. I fiddled with her tablets. Someone, years ago, had diagnosed an underactive thyroid gland, and as she was always tired and sluggish, as well as being enormously overweight, I put her on a dose of thyroxine up to get things going. This gave me something to ask about when I visited.

'Was there any improvement?'

She teased me by offering glimmers of hope.

'A little better doctor, but my bowels are bad'.

So, I gave her bowel mixture. My therapeutic courage began to rise; I experimented with diuretics to release the fluid trapped in her bloated body. Her heart was a bit irregular, so I tried digoxin, a heart stimulant, known for centuries and extracted from the foxglove plant. At last I felt like a real doctor, I was doing something for this unfortunate old lady. By this stage she had me visiting her once a week. A ritual was developing; the care assistant left a teapot ready and two cups. I boiled the tea, examined her while it brewed, and had a quick cup while she told me stories of the past, nearly always related to horses. The encounter would finish with me writing a new prescription for my latest experiment and telling her it was my greatest wish that one day she would be able to go to the chemist to get these herself.

After a while the ritual changed a little, and she began giving me presents. Old cameras of her husband's, tatty old Kodak box cameras. I used to try and refuse them, but she was insistent, a level of guilt began to build up in me, and in the end, I used to pop into the Red Cross Shop across the road with each new acquisition. Then new things were produced, hideous plastic shoehorns with antlers, tacky leather bookmarks, little chrome picture frames etc. The guilt level rose even more, she was buying these things via an intermediary just to keep me coming regularly. Didn't she know I would come anyway, I said to myself. As the realisation of my importance to her very existence began to really impinge on my conscience, I vowed to try to do more with my professional influence. I set a goal in my mind to mobilise Mabel. To get her out of that ghastly little room for a walk in the truly fresh air.

Now every encounter finished not just with a wish but a task, to walk across the room and back, to walk into the back yard etc. She began to respond; a frame was conjured up by the nurses who also became excited by this vision of a mobile Mabel. We professionals now aimed our whole therapeutic force into getting her to go out; it gave us a purpose. I began leading her by the hand across her sticky carpet, the presents stopped but her humour improved. A few years fell away, a light returned to the eyes; she talked of her beloved Elley. For the first time I could actually see her, blond hair streaming, galloping across the Downs. This ruined old lady had been young, vivacious, even attractive, once.

Then came the day. A domiciliary physiotherapist had been working with her for some weeks and was convinced she was ready to try a little journey. As the physio told me this, standing in the back yard, I noticed she was clutching a large plastic shoehorn with antlers. Mabel greeted me enthusiastically:

'I am going to bloody to do it'.

She waited for a reaction; I just smiled and nodded.

'Tomorrow I'm going up the road to the naffing Post Office for me pension. Worked there for twenty year, don't suppose anyone will know me now'.

She mused, and continued:

'That nice girl thinks I should do it so I will'.

She looked at me and I realised that I was not important anymore, that was why the presents had stopped. I should have been happy, but a little touch of pique entered my soul. It grieves me to admit it, but doctors like to be important.

The next morning, while I was seeing patients in my morning surgery, there was an emergency call. Would I go immediately to Abingdon Post Office? My patient Mabel Crump had been involved in a serious accident; the ambulance was standing by. All GPs hate leaving a full surgery; it ruins the day and creates a lot of tension. The story was crystal clear to me already that Mabel had slipped off her frame, twisted her ankle or similar and that this would turn out to be a fuss about nothing. I was irritated too by the feeling that this was my own fault anyway by encouraging this unwise excursion, and naturally arrived at the scene in an unhelpful frame of mind. There was a large crowd outside the Post Office where the ambulance was parked with its blue light flashing. There was another crowd about 50 yards down the road. I parked my car behind the ambulance, waving my stethoscope at the policeman to identify myself (a friend of mine did that once while speeding to an emergency; the policeman waved the handcuffs back). At this time, in the early 1970s, ambulance men were well-trained, but not the protocol-driven, machine-like paramedics of the present day. Doctors were still required at the scene of accidents, although most doctors' training and experience in emergency medicine was none too good. My experience of a busy London casualty department, and a spell as a Ship's Doctor, equipped me better than most. Experience was not needed here; Mabel was dead. She was lying on the pavement, flat on her back, head in a pool of blood and legs characteristically splayed apart. Her eyes were wide and staring though the expression seemed more of wonder than of horror.

'What happened?' I asked inadequately.
'Run over by a horse' said the large, matter of fact ambulance man.

'Sorry, say that again'.

'Yes, a bloody runaway horse, hit her fair and square, look at her frame'.

He pointed at a mangled piece of aluminium tubing some feet away.

'Didn't do the bloody horse any good either, vet's just shot it'.

He gestured to the other gathering down the road. A wave of sadness and uselessness engulfed me, mingled with a feeling that this was just too unbelievable to be true. For five years she had never gone out, and the first time she does she is run over by a bolting horse in the centre of a little market town where there are no horses. A hand touched my sleeve; it was the lady from the Health Food Shop.

'Come with me Doc, I want to show you something'.

The ambulance men took Mabel away to the post-mortem room as a favour to the police whose job it was technically. The butcher took the horse away. I was led into her flat.

'The lady at the Post Office said that she screamed "Elley" just before the horse hit her, I think she thought her old horse had come back for her. Maybe she was right. Here, look here'.

She pulled open a large drawer to reveal bottles of pills going back several years, all unopened.

'She didn't believe in pills'.

She looked at me pityingly.

'Did you like your shoehorn?'

Not long afterwards my father died, from an acute occlusion of the left anterior descending coronary artery. This, as it transpired, turned out to a hereditary weakness. He was 57. I travelled up from the south to help my mother clear out his basement surgery in Beach Road. The smell of damp was strong, a faded print of Landseer's *Monarch of the Glens* was slightly skew-whiff on the mould-covered wall, and it was unutterably gloomy. There were no notes worth the candle, but there was his old microscope, the pestle and mortar, the red, green and brown bottles of non-descript, placebo-laced power, the empty gin bottles, and about five years' worth of the *British Medical Journal*, still in their brown wrappers, piled up on the examination couch. Behind his huge old desk was a little drawer, in which was an open copy of *Tristram Shandy*, and the patient's tatty and rickety chair was placed directly in front of the desk.

My father's funeral at the local crematorium was attended by a larger crowd than the average Sunderland AFC match. So many people I didn't know came up to embrace me (a rare thing for Geordies) and said how much they loved him, but one man stands out in my mind. He sought me out as the crowd was dispersing. He held my hand and looked at me hard.

'Peter, isn't it? And you a doctor, too. Not as good as him, though. Your dad, he was special. He used to listen to you. Didn't examine you much' (I had worked that one out). 'But he listened, and he knew. He always knew, never wrong. Because he always listened, he always knew what mattered'.

This concept of 'mattering' was new to me, and it would have been good to talk to my Dad about it. The concept crystallised not long afterwards when I became ill. I had collapsed twice, once at home and then the next day while consulting. The patient, a female frequent attender, watched me hit the floor, got up and on her way out told the receptionist that Dr Tate was a bit funny. My medical partner found me lying on the floor and I came around to him crying over me, thinking me dead, which was cheering in an odd sort of way. At least he cared. The diagnosis was sick sinus syndrome. My pulse rate had always been around 50 and I had thought, despite my cigarette habit, that it was because I was fit. Ah, hubris.

My pacemaker insertions, firstly in January and again in February 1977, were pivotal moments in many ways. The first insertion was extremely painful; I was told it was a more or less painless procedure. They were fairly new then, and usually inserted into the elderly with poor musculature. I was fit, aged 30, worked out, and had a six pack to be proud of, which was not conducive to pushing a large object, the size of a pack of cards back then, under the tight skin. The light anaesthetic cocktail was totally inadequate but what can you do? I grinned and bore it, but when afterwards, to save others, I told the doctors about the pain, I was dismissed, a wimp, the first one to complain etc. The nurses were more sympathetic, but not much. The hospital experience was unnerving, lonely, but at least short. I was back at work within the week. A couple of weeks later, at home in the early morning, I rolled over in bed and felt unwell, and my chest wall began rhythmically contracting to the beat of my heart. I nudged my wife Sandra who took in the situation very quickly. We decided not to wait for an ambulance and she drove my MGB like a maniac straight to the Old Radcliffe Infirmary. I had enough time to contemplate the imminent tamponade, but it never actually happened. The whole lot had to be done again, quickly and even more painfully. Briefly I was given a single bedded cubicle, but was thrown out after only a few hours. I can tell you the date I had my second pacemaker by looking on Wikipedia, not because I merit an entry but because Anthony Crossland, the senior Labour politician and writer, had a severe cerebral haemorrhage and was admitted on 13th of February 1977. His need was greater than mine, so I was evicted from my cubicle. He died four days later.

As I lay in the old Radcliffe Infirmary, the fear slowly passed to be replaced by an angry emptiness. They kept me in for a week, but nobody wanted to talk to me, no explanations were forthcoming. Perhaps it was because I was a doctor, but after watching and discussing with other patients, the widespread lack of meaningful communication was plain to see. I was beginning to glimpse what really mattered, and I was cross at being old before my time. I never played cricket again.

My death at a young age seemed more probable than not to me, and this realisation focussed my wandering mind. I wanted to be better than I was before I left this life, and was angry at my father for not leaving anything behind. He was a good artist, had several novel insights into Ancient Egypt, but had left no written record and destroyed his paintings as not being good enough. The love of his patients was too transitory for me; he should have made more of a mark. I decided, quite deliberately, to try to make something of my life, but how? I joined the Thames Valley Faculty of the RCGP and met some fun, really sharp doctors, like Theo Schofield, the aforementioned Peter Havelock, Martin Lawrence, John Hasler and Peter Pritchard.

I re-read *The Future General Practitioner* and even understood most of it. But more interesting was the new book by Professor Pat Byrne and his researcher Barrie Long, *Doctors Talking to Patients*. It seemed it was not just hospital doctors who were struggling. Their study of 2,000 audiotaped consultations showed that GPs developed a set of behaviours, and used these stock patterns repeatedly whatever the presenting problem. This remarkable consistency allowed the researchers to categorise doctors according to their style along a scale that they described as doctor-centred to patient-centred. No doctor spanned the whole range; those described as patient-centred showed more flexibility, but overall the impression was of a chastening rigidity. Was I trapped in my own style? To be a more effective doctor I would have to look at my own consulting, recognise my strengths and weaknesses, identify a style and modify it to achieve… to achieve what?

Well, that was the question.

REFERENCES

Balint M. 1957. *The Doctor, His Patient and the Illness*. London: Tavistock Publications.

Byrne PS & Long BEL. 1984. *Doctors Talking to Patients*. Royal College of General Practitioners; Revised edition; January.

Royal College of General Practitioners. 1972. *The Future General Practitioner – Learning and Teaching*. British Medical Journal London.

3

Life Quest

When I first became a trainer in 1977, I was not very good. Not because I didn't know much educational theory, which I didn't, or because I wasn't very well, which I wasn't, but mainly because I was not clear enough about what I did know that might be useful to my marginally more insecure registrar Juliet. She was really cross, having had me foisted on her when my senior partner suddenly jumped ship on a sabbatical to be near his mistress. Staying at my house early on, we did a weekend on-call together. Juliet went to visit a middle-aged lady with chest pain, and came back afterwards for the debrief. The gist of it was that she was an overanxious, recently divorced, chain-smoker who had had a row with her daughter, and Juliet had reassured her and given her a tranquilliser. We went over the clinical symptoms again, myself with increasing unease as this did sound cardiac, even allowing for my current anxiety regarding hearts. Juliet went back, re-looked at this anxious but ill lady, and admitted her with a quite nasty myocardial infarction (MI). During the lady's subsequent cardiac catherisation her main femoral artery was damaged, and her leg gave her intermittent trouble for many years afterwards. This patient and I became close friends over subsequent years, but her ending was a sad one which I will tell you about in Chapter 9, if you get that far. For being a smart arse, I suspect I went down in Juliet's estimation.

I tried to read myself out of trouble. Dennis Pereira-Grey (now Sir) coined the famous triangular trilogy of Aims-Methods-Assessments, hoping that defining the aims of vocational training, or more explicitly the educational needs of GPs, would lead to clear teaching methods that could then be properly assessed. As we all know, it has not turned out to be that easy. The first and major problem was getting trainers to agree on the important aims. This debate rumbled on, and I became a course organiser for the GP vocational training scheme (VTS) in Oxford in 1978. After some years the Thames Valley course organiser group, led by the dynamic John Hasler, tried to more clearly define these aims; an attempted syllabus for the profession. Meanwhile the Leeuwenhorst European Working Party had developed 21 statements, divided into knowledge, skills and attitudes, forming a job description of general practice. Trainer assessment methodologies appeared, the most lasting being the complex Manchester rating scales. No one seemed to agree on what worked best.

In 1979 I had been course organiser in Oxford for a year, and my own inexperience and ignorance of the human condition, let alone teaching ability, was being systematically exposed. I was also still coming to terms with my own mortality, mixed with surprise at how uninvolved in my fears my doctors were; this was my second year with a cardiac pacemaker, and I was just the wrong side of 30. At this uncertain and uncomfortable stage I needed help, and it came quite out of the blue. David Pendleton arrived in my life. A young social psychologist, who exuded passion, drive and necessity. He was saying that doctors should understand their patient's fears, and that communication with patients should be taught as a priority, second only to a good medical education. I wanted this personally, and at last saw a teaching focus and a life quest that I could really engage with. So, like many motives, mine were fundamentally self-centred and, as a result, all the more powerful.

David came to Oxford to do a DPhil on doctor–patient communication. Part of his motivation was to explore the paradox of the poor uptake of medical advice by patients, as described by the so-called 'rule of thirds'. One third of patients take medical advice and act in sufficient accordance with it for the advice to be effective. One third take heed of some of the advice, but not enough for it to be effective. The remaining third just don't bother. Regrettably, this remains the case to this day. David suggested I come to work with him, help him with the DPhil and feed back what we learned to the VTS. In February 1980 I managed to get prolonged study leave and decamped to Oxford for six months.

The Department of Experimental Psychology, the ugliest building in Oxford and rumoured to have been built from the plans of a Bahamian Hotel, was filled with fascinating and terrifyingly intelligent people. Michael Argyll, the doyen of social skills, who would never look you in the eye, the Peters Marsh and Collett, regularly found on television screens, Adrian Furnham the charismatic and very media-friendly soon-to-be professor at University College London, and my favourite, Jos Jaspars, a heavy smoking Dutchman, David's supervisor, and the most clear thinking man I have ever met. He had a model of two mating hedgehogs on his desk. He died only a few years later, far too young. In the adjacent Department of Zoology, the great man-watcher, naked ape and postural echoer, Desmond Morris had his lair. My next-door neighbour and good friend, a Liverpudlian with fierce liberal politics, Geoffrey Ainsley Harrison, Professor of Physical Anthropology, hated Desmond with a passion only true Oxfordian academics can muster, thinking him a fraud, a showman, and a charlatan. I did not have the nerve to tell him that this was possibly just a trifle harsh. Around that time Geoff was the overseer of the Pitt Rivers Museum. Pitt Rivers was a Victorian archaeologist, inveterate collector and colonial plunderer. Geoff took me there late one evening, showing me treasures from Cook's first voyage, a drawer of shrunken heads (tsantsas) and all manner of tribal memorabilia from around the world.

The Department was buzzing, and it was very easy to feel both inferior and out of one's depth, which I did. One morning, early in my stay, a very glamorous, hard-edged Brisbanian called Monica entered our dark, bare, breeze-blocked cell, without so much as a knock. I was conspicuously alone.

'You seen Pendleton?'
'Er no'.
'Know where he is?'
'Er no'.
'Know when he's coming back?'

She looked deep into my ignorant eyes and snorted.

'Jees, I wouldn't pee in your ear if your brains were on fire'.

'Monica doesn't take prisoners' was David's initial contribution.
'I wouldn't like her to criticise my consultations' say I, desultorily shuffling a pile of black and white reel-to-reel videotapes of just that.

'Well it would be a bracing experience,' said David 'but probably not a constructive one; you would need rules'.

This was the seed; how could we discuss something as sensitive, personal and vulnerable as consulting without it turning into a destructive disaster? We kept coming back to this crux. Peter Havelock, a GP in Bourne End near High Wycombe, and Theo Schofield, a GP in Shipston-on-Stour near Stratford, were VTS course organisers too, and all three of us were trying to teach consulting on our respective courses. In the car one day, Bing Crosby sang about accentuating the positive and eliminating the negative; a few conversations and a seminar later we had our rules.

Rule 1: Good points first.
Rule 2: No criticism without recommendation.

The principle was to teach from observed strengths, so building confidence and fostering the creation of a milieu conducive to learning sensitive skills. In young and inexperienced hands like mine, this produced a whole new style of teaching, described by David after watching one of my VTS seminars as 'hitting the learner with the carrot'.

For our sins, we have spent the last four decades dealing with the cynicism that so easily develops. Insincere praise rankles, and everything before the 'but what could you have done better?' question is seen as bullshit. Only integrity, honesty and practice can get rid of this, but experience has confirmed that the rules (or at least an agreed framework for discussion) are crucial. Doctors can be very destructive, and too much discouragement will stop learning in its tracks.

Those early days of good points first were revelatory. After the traditional response to the question of 'what did you do well?', which was a slow flapping motion of the hands with a silent open and closing of the mouth, well-described as the 'Goldfish response', the groups of young doctors were soon spectacularly good at recognising effective skills in their colleagues without, in the vast majority of cases, being insincere or glutinous. Of course, doctors do like being criticised a bit, and they like the sensation of learning spiced with a bit of mustard sometimes, but the environment has to be safe to allow this to happen, and we soon discovered that if we did let the rules relax too much learners were hurt, and the learning suffered. This is still true.

At this time, we had an early Sony black-and-white video camera and a huge Betamax video player, so we started getting our GP friends, trainers and course organisers to videotape some consultations.

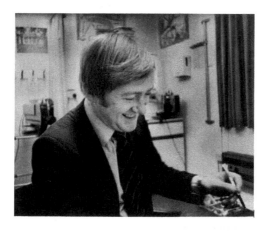

In my surgery in 1979; note the two video cameras.

Then came the hard bit; we began to analyse them, looking for the substance. David interviewed the patients before and afterwards and found that their views of the consultation were not the same as those of the doctor, and often differed markedly from them. Misunderstanding was the norm. Theo Schofield, Peter Havelock, David and I were working closely together by this stage, and we felt that the consultation between doctor and patient needed to be demystified, de-Balinted and the essential tasks clearly delineated. My initial obsession then was studying the use of gestures in the consultation; this set me off mapping events as they happened, and soon this became behavioural mapping of the doctor-patient interaction. Very quickly, I had a hundred or so transparencies of different doctors, including me, consulting. Using Byrne and Long's described behaviours, I could layer several consultations by the same doctor on top of each other. And what do you know? The patterns were strikingly similar, doctors really did do much the same thing in most consultations, including me.

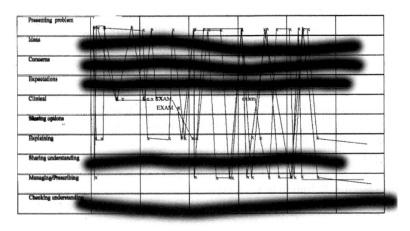

Time in minutes

This is a collection of three of my own consultations, stacked on top of each other to show the consistently absent behaviours at that time.

Around this time, we heard that TV producer Karl Sabbagh and paediatrician Harvey Markovitch were setting up a department to produce educational videos for doctors. We went to London with a proposal to produce such a video based on the GP consultation. They agreed, and having access to the latest cameras and sound recording allowed them to produce GP consultations of broadcastable quality. My partners were somewhat bemused when the team arrived at the Health Centre in Abingdon and recorded two days of my surgeries; the patients were excited and relatively unphased. Others of our friends around the area allowed the cameras in too. David mainly took on the task of editing the material, and with Karl's help produced an extremely fast paced, startling and arresting video programme of GP behaviour in the consulting room. I suppose there might still be a copy in a vault somewhere, but to my shame I don't have one.

The programme began with beginnings and, chasteningly, they were mine. I greeted every patient the same way, yes, everyone, old, young, male, female, posh or oik. 'Hellooo!' says I, ushering my patient to their seat, at least with palpable enthusiasm, which when added together several times approaches Woosterish gormlessness. After a pause of an almost metronomic 10 seconds, the words 'Well now?' with a slight tilt of the head and a poor man's attempt at a raised eyebrow. That was it, my claim to fame, this snippet of ingrained behaviour. When the finished product was released some months later, I began to dread meeting colleagues who would invariably mimic my opening gambit, collapse into laughter and then give me a consoling hug, convinced they were the first ever to have done so. Fame is a very mixed blessing. I grumbled at David for exposing my foibles; he defended himself and curiously me.

'Yours was the best beginning, it is open, non-directive and allows your patient to respond in any way they want. It gives them the control'.

It was certainly a fixed style, I think given to me a decade earlier by John Horder, Balintian to his toenails.

Back in the Department of Experimental Psychology, everyone was seething with attribution theory, promulgated by Gestalt psychologist Fritz Heider, asking why people in various circumstances did what they did. It was just at this moment that fate took a hand. We were sitting drinking coffee in the large open concourse when a very striking young lady walked past. David's head swivelled into a position not normally considered possible, and he immediately made it his business to find out who she was. Jennifer King had come to Oxford to study the Health Belief Model. This interest was serendipitous in so many ways; their subsequent marriage, two daughters and a lifetime working together, being only part. Jenny's clear-headed analysis of the lessons to be learned from this 1950s American social psychological model helped crystallise our thoughts about the consultation.

The Health Belief Model postulates that people's interest in their health and the degree to which they are motivated to change it (*health motivation*) vary enormously. It is the most researched and validated description of patients' beliefs about health and related matters, and it has the following main elements:

Perceived susceptibility: When considering specific health problems, people think very differently about how likely they are to be affected. For example, people who think that they are at high risk of developing lung cancer are more likely to follow advice about giving up smoking than those who do not think they are at risk. If a patient already has a health problem, their perceived vulnerability relates to the degree to which they believe in the diagnosis and its possible consequences. For example, suppose that a patient is diagnosed in the gastroenterology clinic as having irritable bowel syndrome, and it is suggested that tension may be contributing to the condition. If the patient is convinced that pelvic inflammatory disease and not tension is the cause, they are unlikely to adhere to the proposed management plan. This disbelief in what they are told may not be explicit and needs to be searched for. They do not regard themselves as being susceptible to tension, and they therefore conclude that there must be another cause. Their friend was diagnosed with pelvic inflammatory disease and had very similar symptoms, so the doctor must be wrong.

Perceived severity: Patients vary in how dire they believe the consequences of contracting a particular illness or of leaving it untreated would be. Heart disease or lung cancer may seem to be a very remote possibility to a 16-year-old girl who is starting to smoke because of peer pressure. Her attitude may be: 'And anyway by the time I get to 40 they will have a cure for it, won't they?'

On the other hand, the publicity about skin cancer resulting from sun exposure has meant that, in recent years, anxious patients have flocked to doctors with a wide range of minor skin blemishes. Most people regard cancer as very serious, and some, if they suspect it, may even be too frightened to go to the doctor. Particularly sad examples of this, which unfortunately are still not uncommon, include older women with slowly growing fungating carcinomas of the breast. Fortunately, young men with testicular growths do appear to have benefited from the publicity about testicular cancer, and they now seem more likely to attend than was previously the case.

Perceived benefits and barriers: Patients weigh up the advantages and disadvantages of taking any particular course of action. They do not necessarily take all the relevant considerations into account, but they make an evaluation of the perceived costs and benefits nonetheless. This cost–benefit analysis is unique to each individual, and can be influenced by outsiders, including doctors. However, to influence the equation in the patient's favour, those factors that are already included by the patient need to be known by the doctor.

In addition, patients' beliefs do not already exist in a pre-packaged form. They are prompted or created by a number of stimuli and triggers (*cues to action*), such as a physical sensation, what Granny said, what they read online or what has just happened to the man down the road.

The Health Belief Model emphasises that people are generally engaged in a struggle to understand what is happening to them as well as what might happen. Different people try to resolve these dilemmas in different ways. Each person's belief system is of course unique, but it is strongly influenced by race, culture, religion and their immediate society. A poor Chinese farmer will have a very different health understanding to a German banker, but so will people who live in the same environment.

We also discovered that people can be grouped into how they behave when faced by illness. I am talking about 'locus of control', health belief jargon for who or what determines our fate when we are ill. This concept was fashionable at the time, and even now perhaps doesn't get the attention it warrants. Roughly speaking we can divide people into three types. People with an internal locus of control believe they oversee their own health, will listen to trusted advice and are willing to adapt their unhealthy lifestyles. The second type – the fatalist or external controllers – reject most advice except whatever suits their preferences, whereas the third group thinks health is not their responsibility but that of the health professionals. We realised that if the doctor wants to make that crucial connection, the communicative strategy of involvement and sharing that will work for patient A will be much less effective for patient B and probably won't work at all in patient C.

We had learned that to be an effective doctor, it was not enough just to get the clinical part of the consultation right. You had to understand where the patient was coming from and mould your management of their problem to fit in with their belief system. What was more, without discovering every individual patient's health beliefs and checking their understanding, there could be no real participation in the decision-making. To make it easier to teach these insights, we dissected out the now infamous trio of Ideas, Concerns and Expectations (ICE). That mnemonic, ICE, has spawned a thousand courses and much irritation. Nonetheless, the real essence of any effective consultation is for both parties to achieve as genuine a shared understanding as possible. By this time, we knew that this did not happen very often, and was not easy to achieve.

David Pendleton and John Hasler wanted to write an overview of the current important academic thought, and called it *Doctor–Patient Communication*. They contacted many of the top researchers and thinkers of the time, including my hero Professor Pat Byrne, who agreed to write a chapter on doctors' style. I have to be honest here, I never met him. I once saw him across a room at a meeting, but never actually spoke to him. He was a humble Westmoreland GP who had a sudden attack of academia, became a founder member and then, like William Pickles, a leading light in the early RCGP, and became the first English Professor of General Practice at Manchester. He was by all accounts a great raconteur and prodigious Claret drinker. Pat Byrne had just retired when, sadly, in late February 1980 he dropped dead. David, knowing my hero worship, asked me to write his chapter, the full text of which you can find in the Appendix. I concluded in the chapter that individual doctors vary in their style of consulting, with style being a unique blend of behaviours determined by skills and attitudes, and influenced by personality, experience and education. All doctors should be aware of the effects of their ways of behaving on their patients. Most importantly, we should learn that these behaviours are not immutable. We can all, with (a little) help (from our friends), learn new behaviours and skills, possibly bringing about changes in our attitudes. Future training of all doctors must be intimately concerned with the question of style.

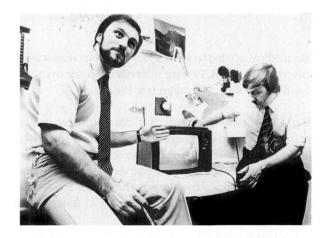

David Pendleton and I reviewing video recordings, 1980.

My sabbatical was halfway through, it was a beautiful Oxford spring in 1980 and David and I were taking a short cut to a meeting via a quiet College garden. There was a glorious medlar in full flower and then we were stopped in our tracks. It was a madrigal, played on a flute, haunting, magical and absolutely no one in sight. We stood, transfixed until it ended, with tears in our eyes. It was Max Beerbohm, friend of Oscar Wilde, who said: 'I was a modest, good-humoured boy. It is Oxford that has made me insufferable'.

By the mid-1980 there were clearly four of us who wanted to develop our thoughts on the learning and teaching of general practice consultations; Theo Schofield, Peter Havelock, myself and of course David. Jenny King, by now girlfriend and imminently fiancée of David, was actively involved, as was John Hasler.

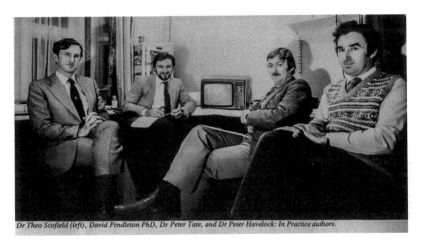

Dr Theo Scofield (left), David Pendleton PhD, Dr Peter Tate, and Dr Peter Havelock: In Practice authors.

David decided we needed to write a book on the consultation, and the Oxford University Press (OUP) were interested. So, for over two years we developed and tested ideas. I wrote in late 1982 that:

Learning and teaching about the consultation is a special interest in Oxford and we have all been helped and galvanised by David Pendleton. The district now has three peripatetic video recording machines and cameras and two practices have their own set-up. This means that each trainee has the opportunity to watch himself consult for at least two weeks in every eight.

Much of this consulting material is reviewed in the practice by trainee and trainer, but on one Tuesday in every month there is a two-hour session in the afternoon devoted to discussing one or two consultations brought by the group members.

This input is reinforced at regional level by the introductory courses organised three times a year. At these three-day residential courses, the trainees are introduced to methods of looking at the consultation and to other teaching methods and are encouraged to accept responsibility for their own learning throughout the year. All trainees attend such a course within two months of starting.

This concentration on the consultation process has been greeted not with resentment but with enthusiasm, but we have needed to develop ways of dealing with potentially explosive and threat-ridden discussions by using rules that insist on always beginning with and concentrating on what is seen to be good. This allows a trust to develop in a group and creates the climate in which subtle and delicate matters can be raised.

We used to meet in the evenings over supper, usually in Oxford, quite often at a little posh restaurant in Summertown, Le Quat' Saisons, run by a chatty little Frenchman who was sometimes hard to understand, called Raymond Blanc. All four of us were strongly opinionated, pig-headed and convinced we were right. It was like four stags competing; there was a lot of head clashing and antler locking. Now none of us can remember who thought of what, but it was a necessary part of the creative process then.

We came up with seven consulting tasks fairly early and honed them via the various groups we ran. They were:

1. To define the reasons for the patient's attendance
2. To consider other problems
3. To choose an appropriate action for each problem
4. To share the doctor's understanding of the problem with the patient
5. To involve the patient in the management of the problem and encourage him to accept the appropriate responsibility
6. To use time and resources appropriately
7. To establish or maintain a relationship with the patient which helps to achieve the other tasks.

Very early on we linked up with the Manchester-based group, North West Spanner, a wonderful group of actors who were brilliant at playing patients and could give doctors very accurate feedback on how effective their consulting skills really were. Our biggest bone of contention was whether it was necessary to teach skills to help doctors complete our seven tasks. The reason we had travelled so far down this pathway was to get away from prescriptive skills training, particularly without clear goals of what to use them to achieve. In the end we decided on a fairly simple list of strategies and skills.

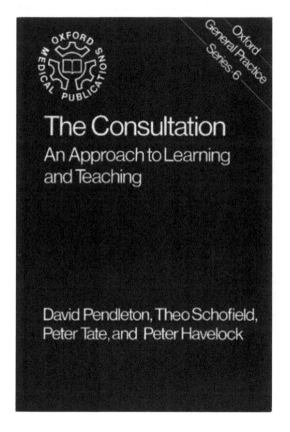

The Consultation: An Approach to Learning and Teaching was published as number six in the OUP Oxford General Practice Series in early 1984. We dedicated the book to Ben Pomryn, a North European psychiatrist who pioneered psychiatry in the community and did his clinics in GP surgeries, usually with a GP sitting in with him. All the real psychiatry I ever knew came from Ben, his perceptive ability was extreme and revelatory, but he did have one fault. He found it hard to stop. He could peel people like they were onions, layer after layer, and sometimes I found my brake foot unconsciously pressing hard against the desk. But on he went, leaving a metaphorically naked soul staring round like a figure in Michelangelo's Last Judgement. We GPs often felt this was too brutal, but Ben would have none of it. He hated wishy-washy reassurance and, in his defence, probably many more of our patients got better because of him than because of me.

By this stage it was clear to me that, while I could be described by a generous friend as a good doctor, it was obvious that I was not a great one. Too impatient, too impetuous and perhaps too trusting. The biggest hole in my leaky repertoire was the ability to understand and help addiction. ICE did not seem to work well, as I never seemed to achieve enough understanding to share. My wife Sandra was by now showing unmistakable signs of alcohol addiction and I was singularly and distressingly not helping her. Meanwhile, Abingdon had its own little explosion of hard drug addiction, mostly heroin. It was winter 1984.

Oscar Black became a patient. Late 20s, handsome if a little gaunt, swept back, slicked, shiny black hair and penetrating, pleading eyes. Quite a striking young man, but his most defining feature was his unglamorous NHS crutches; he had almost total paralysis of both legs from an old accident in South Africa where he had lived for some years. This, among other reasons, was why he was now hopelessly reliant on heroin. He had moved from Jericho, Oxford because the Abingdon drug clinic was considerably more lenient and, on reflection, probably because the GPs were a softer touch. It is only the occasional patient who gets under one's skin; to function there has to be a degree of emotional detachment, but not too much. It is a very fine line to tread. Oscar crossed it for reasons that, even nearly 40 years later, I am unable to explain. He became a mission. I had to help him, to use my hard-learned academic know-how to make his life better. Over a period of months, I saw him far too often, and he shared his hopes and dreams. He was going to set up a little business importing soapstone carvings from his connections in South Africa. I have one still, a grizzled, majestic Negro head in the china cabinet. This soapstone was a far more durable material than the frail glass that contained Oscar's regular prescription of methadone, the ineffective opiate substitute. The variations on a theme would have delighted Paganini, but to my own chagrin usually I gave in and replaced the prescription. I was being played like a violin by a virtuoso.

Sandra and I were members of a local theatre group, and went to Stratford to see Shakespeare's *Richard the Third*, played by rising star Antony Sher. There were rumours that this was a revolutionary production, and that the central performance was electrifying. Well it was, especially to me. The curtain rose, revealing a single figure silhouetted, holding himself up on NHS crutches.

Now is the winter of our discontent
Made glorious summer by this son of York;
And all the clouds that lour'd upon our house
In the deep bosom of the ocean buried.

It was Oscar, or so it seemed to me; for a period of minutes I actually believed it was and found myself constructing all sorts of unlikely fantasies to explain the inexplicable. At the interval I tried to explain my copious tears away but what could I say? Sandra was convinced I had the problem, not her. As we drove home, we passed an outdoor shop with a brightly lit sign saying, and I swear this is true, 'Now is the Winter of our Discount Tent'.

After that extremely strange experience I saw Oscar differently; Shakespeare's Tudor propaganda had seeped into my soul, and I was harder on him and stopped letting him out-manoeuvre me. After a while he went back to Jericho where he died, but not for another 15 years. At least he is not resting under a car park in Leicester.

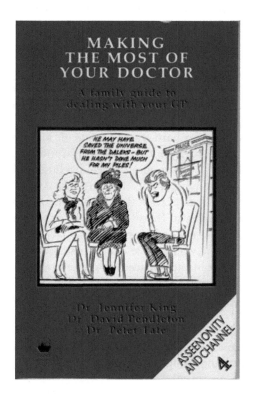

By 1985 Jennifer King and David were married. With Jenny's encouragement and connections, we decided to rewrite *The Consultation*, but for patients this time. We called it *Making the Most of Your Doctor: A Family Guide to Dealing with Your GP*. It was linked to a curious ITV/ Channel 4 sitcom *The Setbacks*, and our episode was *Doctor's Orders*. I think I probably have the only surviving copy. It had cartoons and was full of lists to help patients recognise the sort of doctor they had and the sort of patient they were. I produced several of these lists from a hospital bed as another pacemaker wire had snapped and the system needed rebooting.

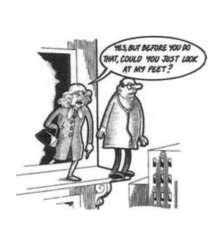

All doctors have off days.

Just one glass a day.

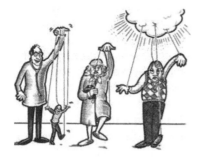

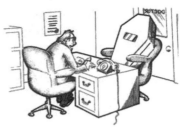

Who's in control of your health?   I hope it wasn't anything urgent.

The book was a minor success, sold over 5,000 copies and hit the national press. The Daily Mail went with '*Patients in fear of bossy doctors*' and the Telegraph with '*A prescription is GP's way of telling you to go*'.

In January 1986, *Pulse* carried the following review:

A simple guide to help people choose a good GP says patients should look for a doctor who has the MRCGP.

The guide – 'Making the Most of Your Doctor' by GP Dr Peter Tate, and social psychologists Dr Jennifer King and Dr David Pendleton – also makes College Fellows a preferred choice because of their 'outstanding service to general practice'.

The booklet published last week, provides a checklist for the patient to work through to eliminate the doctors who are not sufficiently accessible, do not practice prevention, are not good listeners, and practice from 'grotty premises'.

Dr Tate, Dr King and Dr Pendleton, who helped GPs learn how to audit their work when he was Stuart Fellow of the RCGP, have applied the RCGP's "What Sort of Doctor?" method of judging GPs to guide patients in the same task.

This assessed the doctor for accessibility, clinical competence, capacity to communicate and professional values. In the section on clinical competence – 'does the doctor know his stuff?' – the first question the patient should ask is: 'Is your doctor a Member or Fellow of the RCGP?' In the section on ability to communicate, potential patients are advised to ask: 'Does your doctor let you decide with him how your problem should be handled?' Dealing with specialist qualifications a GP might possess, the guide says that if the doctor has the FRCS 'You might wonder why he is in general practice at all'. It also warns patients that if the doctor has MRCVS after his name, he is a vet.

In systematically setting out to choose a doctor, patients are advised to draw up a list of what they want and then visit all the practices near enough to see how they measure up. Practices which have doctors prepared to discuss the sort of care they give to help the patient decide if they want to sign on are preferred. The booklet also guides people in deciding whether a doctor is authoritarian or 'a sharing doctor'.

Patients are warned that most doctors have 'off days', but that if their GP always seems to be having an 'off day' this is cause for concern.

In this book we were trying to help patients make informed choices about the sort of doctor and the sort of communication they should be looking for. This was very much in line with some of the better parts of the upcoming White Paper *Promoting Better Health* (published in 1987 but set in motion in 1985). In some parts of the country, groups had been formed to train patients to communicate effectively with doctors.

A further reason for writing this little book was the hope that actively involved patients would change medical behaviours. We wondered why doctors were so reluctant to involve their patients in their own healthcare. It seemed there must be several reasons, but the crucial one was training. Medical schools took the caring cream of our education system and after five years had turned most of these young idealists into rigid, hidebound, authoritarian tellers; the sharing and the listening had been removed. Another reason was the communication skills doctors possessed. Byrne and Long, as mentioned in Chapter 2, had demonstrated that most doctors had a very limited capacity to change consulting styles when required by the differing needs and types of patients, and we, along with others like David Tuckett's team, were confirming this daily. Each one of us only had a limited range of behaviours at our disposal, which in turn affected our attitudes. We began to think that if a doctor was no good at, or untrained in, say, sharing decision-making, they were likely to ignore such opportunities in the consultation and rationalise it to have a low level of priority. If they then learned the appropriate skills, then the attitude perhaps would be more likely to change to a far more positive one. Yet another hidden reason for keeping patient involvement to a minimum was the threat posed to the doctor. This threat could be the risk of exposing ignorance, of being found wanting, of losing status and power, of increasing our own anxiety levels unacceptably and of using too much precious time. In this book we were certainly waving the College Flag; as it turned out, just a tad too vigorously.

It is not just Quantum Theory that is filled with strange entanglements, life is too. In 1957 my father drove from South Shields to Lloret de Mar on the Costa Brava in a smoke-filled Ford Zephyr, with me on the back seat listening to Eartha Kitt on a small portable Grundig tape recorder. There we met his friend and fellow GP John McKee and his family who were, unlike us, staying at the posh hotel. John was a big, affable, slightly frightening man, a magistrate and perpetual optimist, being the long-term prospective Tory candidate for South Shields. John's son Ian was a few years older than I and made it plain that, to him, I was an irritating little squirt. He was probably right. Our lives rarely intersected after that, though my parents always related news of his doings. He became a GP in Edinburgh and we lost what little touch we had ever had until *Making the Most of Your Doctor* was published.

In 1986 Ian was senior partner in a large practice, and editor of *The Physician*, a trade magazine for GPs with a title suggesting it was somewhat grander than it actually was. He had for years harbored a dislike of the RCGP and had never joined himself. Fair enough, I was only a relatively recent convert, but he was very cross at the suggestion that one way to choose a GP was by degree, especially the MRCGP (Membership of the Royal College of General Practitioners). He wrote the leading editorial *The Physician* in April 1986 titled '*Should the RCGP be reported to the GMC*'. At the time, there were valid reasons for this doubt, as many MRCGP doctors then had not taken the examination. He took the view that our College Flag waving was in fact denigrating non-members, and a serious slur on their reputations. He went as far to suggest that I, as the sacrificial lamb of the RCGP, be referred to the GMC. The Chairman of the GMC Committee on the Standards of Professional Conduct and Medical Ethics at the time was Donald Irvine (also very recently RCGP Chair), of whom more to come.

This spat must be seen in the context of the time. General practitioners, since the birth of the NHS, were paid per capita, and so income depended on the number of patients registered on their list. This led to local competition, rivalry and, in some cases, patient-poaching, such as during an acrimonious partnership split. To some extent, vestiges of this remain to the present day, but different payment methods and decreasing numbers of GPs have led most modern GPs to want fewer patients rather than more. Even by 1986 this was much less of an issue, and the row blew over relatively quickly. A short article in *Doctor* sums it up:

The RCGP has angrily rejected a suggestion that it be reported to the GMC for unethical conduct because of claims in a booklet that College members make better GPs than other doctors.

Among the doctors acknowledged for ideas contributed on how to choose a good doctor are Dr John Hasler, RCGP Council Chairman, and College luminaries Prof David Metcalfe and Dr Theo Schofield.

Dr McKee writes: 'If this booklet achieves the success its publishers desire, it means that members of the RCGP will be more successful in recruiting new patients than non-College members; their income will rise as a consequence'.

And he invites objectors to alert the GMC Committee on the Standards of Professional Conduct and Medical Ethics, the chairman of which is Dr Donald Irvine, immediate past chairman of the RCGP council.

Dr Tate said he would be delighted to appear before the GMC to defend himself. He claimed that Dr McKee had taken *his suggestions out of context. While he said the MRCGP qualification was a valid criterion for choosing a good doctor, he had also listed about 30 other criteria, including accessibility and premises.*

Dr Hasler said: 'I provided general information about what patients should look for; it did not include the MRCGP'.

I was never summoned to the GMC, although I did write to Ian, who wrote back saying that at least he had bought a copy, and his mother was in fear of being ejected from the South Shields golf club bridge circle.

Around this time the then Chief Examiner Andrew Belton wrote to The Times.

A couple of years later I wrote *'Burned out or just disillusioned?'* describing how the VTS course's mission to bring to post-graduates the desire to look at, learn from and think about all aspects of general practice was being increasingly questioned by trainees. My 'special evangelism' for the study of communication between doctor and patient was now being perceived by trainees in the same way as they saw all aspects of 'behavioural' medicine, as peripheral to the nitty-gritty, day-to-day exercise of tried, but not very tested, clinical skills. Like many of us who taught general practice, I clearly believed that the doctor fresh from hospital needed re-educating. However, the trainees felt that they still needed educating, and perhaps that was the nub of the problem.

The trainee had not been taught, either in medical school, clinical training or hospital jobs, the basic clinical communication skills that are clearly needed in general practice. There was a 'wind of change' in the minds of both the assessor and assessed.

The possession of certain clinical communication skills had been neglected, or rather had taken too unimportant a place, for too long.

REFERENCES

Byrne PS & Long BEL. 1976. *Doctors Talking to Patients*. London: HMSO.

King J, Pendleton D & Tate P. 1985. *Making the Most of Your Doctor*. London: Thames Methuen.

Pendleton D & Hasler J. 1983. *Doctor–Patient Communication*. London: Academic Press.

4

The American Adventure

The publication of *The Consultation: An Approach to Learning and Teaching* in 1984 gave David, Peter, Theo and myself a degree of street cred, and entry into a different circle of friends. One of these new friends was David Smith, a Professor of Human Values at the University of South Florida (USF). Dave was quick-witted, acerbic and enthusiastic about our mission to empower patients. His field was medical ethics and he liked gladiatorial verbal contests, as well as the Tampa Bay Buccaneers, an NFL team of a similar stature and ineptitude to my own beloved Sunderland AFC. We formed a bond and he asked me to come to America to 'learn how it is really done'. I was given a substantial grant from the Claire Wand fund and my family packed its bags. My GP partners were fed up, off again! Before we left, we had a party in late August to celebrate my upcoming 40th; a Christmas party with turkey, crackers and Christmas pud, as we would be across the pond for the real event. The best bit of the party was throwing buns from the balcony of our little cottage in Culham; it was mayhem. This was based on the time-honoured, if daft, Abingdon custom of the Council throwing buns from Christopher Wren's County Hall to the hoi polloi below. My daughter Elizabeth, now in her 40s, says it is the most memorable event of her childhood.

I kept a diary of our American adventure. Early in September 1986 my wife Sandra and I, with our children Elizabeth, six, and Richard, five, flew from Heathrow, changed at Miami (a chastening experience) and arrived in Tampa. Jeanne, Dave's wife, was there holding a large placard labelled TATES, and greeted us with real warmth. Her Dodge convertible had no front number plate, the handbrake was weird and the lane discipline very un-English. The strangeness was good. We stopped for a burger and the waitress said 'You're welcome, you got it, have a nice day'. I asked for a beer instead of the coke. 'My we have a drinker in here tonight'.

We were given a condo in Clearwater with a swimming pool, fishing pier and a lake out to the back and sea out to the front. The kids thought they had gone to heaven.

We were invited to Dave and Jeanne's for an early evening BBQ, the first gas one I had ever seen. Just as dusk fell there was an explosion of sound; katydids, the American cicada and very loud. The trees were covered in what looked like tissue, like something straight out of Miss Havisham's bedroom; this was Spanish moss, a sort of air plant. Dave sagely advised me not to touch the stuff; 'full of red bugs, chiggers, little buggers will bite you all over, especially where you don't want them'.

A wonderful 80-year-old car salesman, Wilson Records, rented me a 1984 Oldsmobile Cutlass Supreme for $250 a month. It was like driving a bath. He gave me a plastic pink flamingo to seal the deal. I learned from Dave that this was the symbol of extreme tackiness in Florida; there was a shop that sold nothing else.

David had a contract to instill improved communication and ethical thinking into the Department of Family Medicine at USF. It was not going too well. Dave's big champion, the Dean of USF had left suddenly, and it turned out that the family doctors were, at best, lukewarm. Dave was hoping that my presence might galvanise developments in his favour. Spoiler alert, it didn't.

To begin with, we visited Bayfront Medical Centre and met some of the family physicians there; they confided that family physicians and specialists had a poor relationship. They also worried that American medical schools turned out scientists interested in diseases, and not people. Much the same the world over I mused to myself. I met several members of the Department; they were all friendly, and most said they wanted to invite us to various gatherings. I felt welcomed, but Dave poured cold water on my favourable impressions; 'You might get one or two invites, but they won't ask you back, trust me'. He turned out to be right. The American family physicians were superficially friendly but cold underneath; they said all the right things, but invitations didn't quite happen. I asked Dave why, was it me? Probably he replied, but my real problem was that I didn't do American Christianity; they had me sussed as an unbeliever, so they wouldn't let me into their kingdom. It was a theory, but looking back I did feel a bit lonely.

What expertise I had to offer was in the dissection of doctors' consulting behaviour. I was by this time quite skilled in video tutorials, and well experienced in leading groups of young doctors. There was an embryonic video department and it was suggested that I helped to get this up and running. This was something I could get my teeth into and I agreed with some enthusiasm. After four months I had managed one session.

The equipment never worked; the technician always almost fixed it. On the rare occasions it did work, prearranged sessions or meetings just did not happen. It took a long time to dawn on me, but the Department just did not want this sort of 'intrusion'. Dave was seen as an abrasive nuisance, and I was seen as a foreign interloper.

I was allowed to run seminars on consulting theory and gave talks on developments in communication. These seemed well received, but hands-on consulting teaching was definitely off of the agenda. The most well-attended talks were on the NHS, about which they were curious, but there was a universal, ingrained distrust, even dislike, of 'socialised medicine', and although in England I had had several doubts about our system, viewed from across the pond its successes far outweighed its faults. They were fascinated at my defence of an, in their view, indefensible system. There were one or two heretics, but they whispered to me in private and trusted me to keep their confidence.

Overall, the family doctors and their trainees were not happy with their lot. They felt their lessened status in the profession, and many had heavy workloads to pay the bills. Several were moonlighting in the Emergency Room (ER) at Bayfront Hospital. As one said to me, 'it is not the emergencies and that sort of stuff that gets to you, it is the daily getting pecked to death by ducks that does it'.

Then I met a real, non-academic, family doctor. Malcolm was my age, English, qualified in Leeds and drove a Porsche Carrera. He and his wife had two children of similar ages to mine, and they all lived in a mansion with sea views. We quickly struck up a friendship and he took me on a typical day in his working life. First, we went to the Suncoast Medical Clinic. This big building, which Malcom owned 10% of, was smart, modern and well equipped. Around 40 doctors worked here, of various specialties, but the GPs owned it. Malcolm employed a secretary to take the patient's histories. The patients were all waiting in green paper pyjama tops. Malcolm glanced at the history proforma, did the most cursory examination and the conversation was mainly non-medical, more encouraging and 'matey'. He asked a young man recovering from 'flu to come back in a week. Why I asked? Because he's insured! Of course, how stupid of me. I surreptitiously timed the encounters, most lasted about three minutes, with a range of between one and seven minutes. I could not use a consultation map to dissect these interactions because there was nothing to map. I began to get a glimmer of understanding as to why the Department of Family Medicine did not want me anywhere near them with a video recorder. Malcolm explained to me, as to a dim child, that the GP wants their patient to get well at maximum profit, and to like him enough to come back frequently. There was no incentive to keep the patient healthy, and there was an imperative to refer for investigations and second opinions because that was how the system worked, and what patients expected. The 'preventive leaflets' scattered in profusion all over the building were in fact selling a range of costed check-ups that kept the system fed; mammograms, flexible sigmoidoscopies, chest x-rays, CT scans etc. The dietary health messages were there to sensitise people about their health, stimulating introspection that might lead to further consultations. Patients wanted 'health' via payable bills, quick service, civility and getting what they wanted. I was feeling uncomfortable.

We drove on to Humana Hospital Sun Bay where Malcolm looked after a group of long-term inpatients. It was soon apparent that many patients were 'mentally incompetent', disorientated or absolutely gaga. I think of Sam Shem's *House of God*, to which we will return. Shem coined the word GOMER, a shortened version of Get Out of My Emergency Room. These GOMERS were being treated very intensively, and professionally, with no clinical stone left unturned. For what? I ask. Malcolm told me that it was their constitutional right. There could be no discrimination on race or creed (bullshit; what really mattered was their insurance package) and that legally they had to do everything. I was naively horrified that this sort of medicine was an academic game of electrolytes and other blood parameters, fluid charts and hyperalimentation. If there was any doubt, a referral was made; Malcolm made several on our visit. Its purpose was to do everything that someone, later, might say you should have done. It was also mad, inhuman and grossly unkind, and couldn't be 'ethical' in any reasonable understanding of the word. I vowed, there and then, never to work in America.

Malcolm used the SOAP (an acronym for subjective, objective, assessment and plan) system as a method of writing out notes in a patient's chart. This documentation of patient encounters in the medical record was an integral part of practice workflow, starting with patient appointment scheduling, through writing out notes, to medical billing. You wouldn't have found ideas, concerns and expectations in this system. It was explained that all of these admissions, referrals and treatments were overseen by a Peer Review Organisation (PRO), established by the Tax Equity and Fiscal Responsibility Act of 1982 to review quality of care and appropriateness of admissions, readmissions and discharges for Medicare and Medicaid. These organisations were held responsible for lowering admission rates, reducing lengths of stay (how ironic), while insuring against inadequate treatment. PROs could conduct reviews of medical records and claimed to evaluate the appropriateness of the care provided. I may be cynical, but I think they only worked to the benefit of the established doctors who could pull the strings.

To return to Sam Shem, the pen name of the American psychiatrist Stephen Joseph Bergman, whose main books *The House of God* and

Mount Misery are fictional but close-to-real, first-hand descriptions of the training of doctors in the United States. By chance I was reading *The House of God* at this time. It is a must-read; funny, insightful, brutal and very sad. Among the most memorable bits are his rules for surviving as an ER doctor in a large hospital:

> GOMERS don't die. GOMERS go to ground.
> At a cardiac arrest, the first procedure is to take your own pulse.
> The patient is the one with the disease. Placement comes first.
> There is no body cavity that cannot be reached with a #14G needle and a good strong arm.
> They can always hurt you more.
> The only good admission is a dead admission.
> If you don't take a temperature, you can't find a fever.
> Show me a BMS (Best Medical Student, a student at The Best Medical School) who only triples my work and I will kiss his feet.
> If the radiology resident and the medical student both see a lesion on the chest x-ray, there can be no lesion there.
> The delivery of good medical care is to do as much nothing as possible.

This last rule was being totally ignored in Florida in 1986.

Malcolm took me to a lunchtime lecture on depression by a female psychiatrist with frizzy hair. 'How do you differentiate depression from human unhappiness?' I asked at the end. 'If they are unhappy longer than three weeks I give 'em pills' she replies.

I thought I was beginning to understand, but I was wrong. I tried to debrief with Dave that afternoon, expecting confirmation of my feelings and some empathy. This was a mistake; he became defensive, telling me how good American medicine was, how it was much fairer than I thought it, and far, far, better than the dozy system that existed in the UK. I had taken up jogging and went for a long one that evening, down by the huge, pink Don Cesar Hotel, past the Hurricane restaurant, famed for its grouper burgers, and along Pass-a-Grille Beach. It was a glorious sunset.

Somewhat shaken, the next day I returned to the Department of Family Medicine; a resident was introducing the morning lecturer. 'Doctors prescribe drugs about which they know little, to cure illnesses about which they know less, to human beings about whom they know nothing. Well today we have a guy who knows a lot about human beings, Dr Charles Culver, and he will enlighten us about living wills'. Dr Culver urged us to encourage our patients to think about what they wanted, and the situations in which they would want to refuse certain treatments. He encouraged the audience to fill in their own living will. I wondered if the Humana Hospital would be keen on Dr Culver.

Charles Culver was a well-known, premier league ethicist, and the residents had been asked to bring some difficult cases for discussion. A week or so before, I had met a poor little girl called Patti in her lonely hospital bed, and her case was presented by the chief resident. Patti was 18-month old, Black, and had already been in hospital for five months, admitted with a *Pneumocystis carinii* chest infection, and had active, congenital AIDS. Her dad had died of it, and her mum was HIV positive. Patti was sick a lot, and so was fed intravenously, and barrier-nursed. One hour a day, hired for that purpose, a play therapist played with her, while wearing a face mask and gloves. Patti was dying, very slowly, and endured regular blood tests to measure her platelets, electrolytes and so on. She was on a barbiturate to stop any seizures, and antibiotics to check the infection. She was, unsurprisingly, terrified of people in white coats.

The chief resident, Patti's doctor, believed in control; everything in his control should be done. The Ethics Committee had been very wishy-washy. Only Patti's assigned nurse thought that they were all a bunch of arrogant bastards and refused to come to the case conference. I had drawn a cartoon and written a poem, while crying, the day that I saw Patti. After the presentation Dave, who has seen it, asks me to read it out.

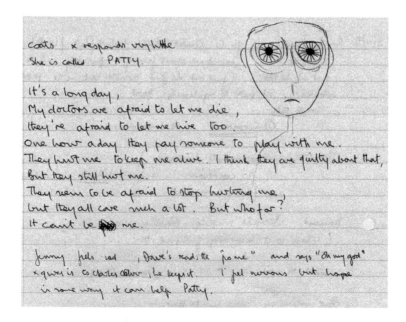

coats × responds very little
She is called   PATTY.

It's a long day,
My doctors are afraid to let me die,
they're afraid to let me live too.
One hour a day they pay someone to play with me.
They hurt me to keep me alive. I think they are guilty about that,
but they still hurt me.
They seem to be afraid to stop hurting me,
but they all care such a lot. But who for?
It can't be me.

Jenny feels sad, Dave's read the "poem" and says "Oh my god"
× quesi is to Charles Culver, he keeps it. I feel nervous but hope
in some way it can help Patty.

Patti
It's a long day
My doctors are afraid to let me die.
They are afraid to let me live too.
One hour a day they pay someone to play with me.
They hurt me to keep me alive. I think they are guilty about that.
But they still hurt me.
They seem to be afraid to stop hurting me.
But they all care such a lot. But who for?
It can't be me......

The chief resident refused to talk to me. It was going well, this American trip. He talked about AIDS treatments, and said he did not wish to look after AIDS patients. This is a professional decision. A committed Christian physician commented that 'it's a whole new ball game now they say it can be heterosexually spread; before it was just those homos and indigents'. No one talked of compassion. Paul, the medical student, said he examined his two AIDS patients without wearing gloves to make them feel human, and liked to talk with them, but can't tell his colleagues for fear of ridicule. The main discussion centres around the best ways of saying no to patients. That evening I go for another long jog; I get a lot of extrasystoles.

The next day a hitherto quiet, earnest, older doctor pulled me into a quiet room and shut the door. 'Englishman, I don't think you will have seen real ignorance till you came down here to downtown St Pete' he said to me, 'but you ain't been to Baton Rouge yet. In Baton Rouge if they've got sugar diabetes, they expect to have their toes cut off. No cure, no diet, nuthin, but they know their toes'll go. Jees they are so stoopid. And this it isn't racialism, it's a fact. There is nuthin' stoopider than a stoopid black, 'cept maybe a Puerto Rican'. I began to want to go home; certainly to leave.

He had something else he wanted to tell me. 'You want to know about communicating with patients, what about not communicating? Have you heard of the Tuskegee experiment?' He tells me this was sponsored by the US Government, and began in 1932 in Alabama, using a group of 600 Black sharecroppers. Of these 600, 399 of the men had syphilis and 201 were uninfected control patients. Treatment was supposed to be a part of the study, but the Public Health Department had decided to leave the men untreated, and follow the course of the disease to these men's eventual deaths. The poor suckers thought they were receiving an experimental treatment for 'bad blood' in exchange for free meals and a $50 death benefit. However, the study was actually designed to measure the progression of untreated syphilis, and to determine if the natural course of the disease was different in Black men versus white men. By 1947, penicillin had become the standard treatment of syphilis, but the men were never advised that they had syphilis. The original study was only meant to last between six and nine months, but in fact continued for 40 years ending in 1972, long after wives and children had been infected, and many of the men had died of syphilis. It eventually ended because of a story printed in the Washington Star. At the end of this tale he stared at me; to this day I don't know if he was for or against.

I was now nervous about debriefing with Dave and kept the last episode for my diary, but I did tell him I was reading, and finding interesting, Eric Cassells' *Talking with Patients: The Theory of Doctor–Patient Communication*. Dave doesn't like him, telling me that his students gave this book a 70% thumbs down.

We spend Thanksgiving at Dave and Jeanne's. It is wonderful, alcohol loosens tongues and Jeanne confided that she was a psychotherapist who has sort of lost her faith; 'after 20 years I reckoned just telling people to pull themselves together was quickest and probably the best I could do'. Dave told me there were fundamental problems with our task-based consultation model. He said 'we have to unpack this'; a singularly American academic phrase, which in fact means to add on to the simple and concise to make it even more meaningful, which sounded like obfuscation to me. But that was harsh, and he was right. He thought our main weakness was that we had deliberately shied away from offering the skills to achieve the seven tasks set out in *The Consultation*. He dismissed my anxiety about being too prescriptive in skills training, saying 'well, we know some behaviours work well, and some don't; you must be specific when telling people how to improve, you must tell them how'. In the background Berlin were singing 'Take My Breath Away', the theme from *Top Gun*, and the most played tune in Florida at that time. Dave said that he and Jeanne were going to write a book for patients, to skill them for dealing with the system; I hope he has better luck than we did with *Making the Most of Your Doctor*; he didn't.

We visited Chicago, which was very cold, and stayed with Paul and Martha Arntson in Evanston, Cook County. Paul was a Professor of Speech and Communication at North Western University. They were a wonderful family. Paul was a social activist, committed Christian and all-round good guy. His mantra was that for every one part talking, take three parts listening. He lived by his own rules. I was booked to run a few seminars and talk on 'Patient Empowerment', which went well. We liked Chicago and visited the circus, the National History Museum, and travelled on the 'L' (elevated railway). This was particularly exciting as I was just finishing *Cider House Rules* by John Irving. We went up the John Hancock Building, and wandered round a Christmassy Macy's.

Paul highlighted his thoughts on the failures of *The Consultation* approach. There was no menu of skills, so we got stuck, never got to the next level and so frustrated the learners. He felt that 2,000 years of medical tradition was against us. He rejected the patient-centred approach as a load of crap; in his view it was a professional cop-out, and not truly feasible. What mattered was the professional bottom line, what criteria did we doctors use to draw the patient agenda line? Unlike Dave, he believed this had to be a negotiation, not a persuasion, but their views are more similar than disparate.

The kids cried when we left to go back to Florida. Dave had been away too; we met him at his home. He was cross with Jeanne; the swimming pool was green as she had forgotten to add the chemicals. 'Gee when I get home, I expect to mow the lawn not the pool'.

I was allowed a two-day, self-indulgent, solo pilgrimage to San Antonio and the Alamo, a childhood obsession extended into adulthood, which curiously did not disappoint. In the Mission there were medical books belonging to John Purdy Reynolds, a young doctor from Tennessee, who went with David Crocket and a few others to find a new life in Texas. He was running from something and ended up hiding in the middle of a battlefield. I mean to write a story about him, but have not, yet.

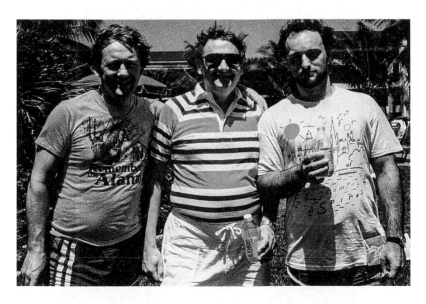

Me, David Smith and David Pendleton Florida 1986.

We went to Disney World in early December and made the mistake of going back on Christmas Day, having been told it will be the quietest day of the year; most of Florida was there. It was horrendous. At the end of the day we got to Cinderella's Castle and met the beautiful, porcelain-featured but exhausted girl of the same name. She advised us to abandon Boxing Day in Disney and go to Sea World instead. We took her good advice. I noted she was not wearing glass slippers.

It was time to go home. We had had good times, but were all looking forward to England in February. I went back on my own for a week in 1988, but never since.

The Americans, years later, did give all four of us an award. Theo went to collect it.

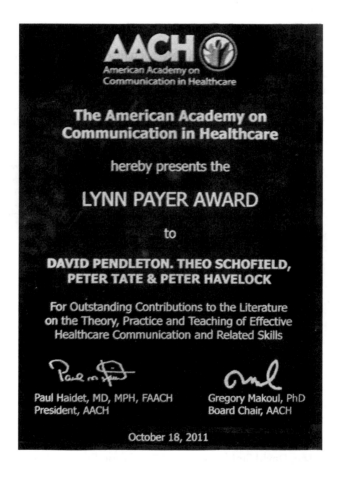

REFERENCES

Cassell E. 1985. *Talking with Patients: Volume 1: The Theory of Doctor–Patient Communication*. The MIT Press.

King J, Pendleton D, & Tate PHL. 1985. *Making the Most of Your Doctor*. Thames-Methuen.

Pendleton D, Schofield T, Tate P et al. 1984. *The Consultation: An Approach to Learning and Teaching*. Oxford: Oxford University Press.

Shem S. 1978. *The House of God*. New York: Dell Publishing.

5

The RCGP

After my time on sabbatical with David Pendleton, I enjoyed working with patients more. For a while I became obsessed by health beliefs and, even now, like to collect the really odd ones. I had learned that nearly 100% of people act reasonably and rationally based on what they believed about health and illness. What I had also learned was that most of these beliefs were unscientific, wishful thinking, bizarre and irrational, including some of my own; that drinking copious amounts of red wine would improve my heart disease, and eating a lot of leeks would cure my gout. Sadly, after prolonged trials, there was a lack of evidence for either. A couple of patient favourites: the lady who loved her 'Aquarius' cream (she meant aqueous) for her psoriasis; 'It works because I am Gemini, and we are very influenced by Aquarius' she told me, with not a trace of irony. Or the nuclear scientist who was convinced that his intermittent atrial fibrillation was directly related to the amount and type of beer he drank, and kept detailed graphs of the correlation, while not altering his drinking habits one jot. He turned up with the graphs in quadruple colours every month for inspection.

An example of a crucial, life-threatening health belief was a young diabetic mother patient at my surgery with two teenage children. She was apparently very conscientious about looking after her diabetes, but her sugars fluctuated wildly, as did her weight. She was initially adamant that she stuck rigidly to her diet. Over several consultations the truth gradually emerged, and it was complex. Her marriage had failed; she was a single working mother with a high-pressure job, and a need to keep up appearances by looking attractive. She knew from her own experience that if her sugar was high for a period of time, she would lose weight and, in her conviction, look more attractive, be more likely to find another partner, and so be happier. But equally significant was her fear of long-term diabetic complications, her real need to keep her sugar levels within a reasonable range, which in her deep-rooted belief meant that her weight had to be controlled at all costs. This belief led to the absolutely paradoxical behaviour of secret chocolate binge-eating, to raise her sugar levels and so lose weight; she believed that such an irrational activity could in fact make her slim and attractive, and so increase her confidence and self-esteem which were directly linked to the achievement of her personal happiness. Only by dissection of these beliefs could she be helped to achieve satisfactory diabetic control and a weight she could accept. The key to finding all of this out was picking up a few cues and following them like a dogged detective, probing and using the knowledge gained about her social and psychological circumstances, then searching out her deeply hidden (from health professionals and some even from herself) health beliefs. In the light of these newly exposed beliefs we were then, and only then, able to negotiate a treatment and management plan which allowed us both to work on a useful and effective treatment regime.

Around this time, I was fascinated by anthropological beliefs about the new disease of HIV and AIDS and what, if anything, could be done to improve things. Many of these beliefs were unpleasant, as well as wrong. For example, many central and southern African males were convinced that having sex with a virgin would cure AIDS by transferring it to her. Apart from being medieval (the same belief about syphilis was common in Europe in the sixteenth century), stupid and dangerous, the effect that this belief was having on families was terrible. Small girls were being raped; families torn apart while the infection was spreading remorselessly. Caribbean men believed they could tell who had AIDS just by looking, and that they could not get an erection with an HIV-positive woman. In New Guinea they buried children alive if they were suspected of having the disease. The African tribes had developed other beliefs about 'the wasting disease' and even the Ngangas (medicine men) had to adapt fast as this was outside of their experience too. Most of the tribes did not think conventional medicine had anything to offer. Sadly, they were right, as no one would pay for retroviral treatment at that time, but their traditional treatments were just pissing in the wind too. The president of South Africa, Thabo Mbeki, publicly denied that HIV caused AIDS; the resulting scientific outcry led to the Durban Declaration in 2000, signed by 5,000 scientists, published to coincide with the International AIDS Conference in Durban that year. Many poor, American whites heavily stigmatised those with AIDS as drug-taking, promiscuous faggots. In some religious quarters it was seen as a disease sent by a wise God to eliminate the undesirables in the society. I saw suggestions of that view during my time in Florida. All in all, most early health beliefs associated with AIDS were pretty nasty, very unhelpful and highlighted the very worst ingrained survival instincts of the human animal.

More recently, worldwide health beliefs about immunisation have allowed previously controlled diseases to regain a foothold; humans instinctively tending towards a perceived non-interventionist, low-risk strategy, seen by the scientifically driven as bizarre. The fact that this has often been driven by rebel professionals makes the countering of these beliefs so much harder.

From coal-face family medicine and life experience, I had learned that people tended towards advice that confirmed, rather than refuted, what they currently believed. Daniel Kahneman later encapsulated this as part of his System One thinking, and called it *confirmation bias*. This new quest made consulting fun in a completing-a-crossword-puzzle sort of way. A person's health beliefs were a clear path to their understanding, and turned formulaic health messages into bespoke consulting. I listened a lot more and tried to nudge rather than direct. Hippocrates might chuckle, Osler too, and my Dad. They knew this instinctively, without having to wade through hours of video recording, but to me it was life-changing and enhancing. I like to think it helped some of my patients too. And at last I really understood what mattered. It was unique for everyone, but to discover it all you had to do was to be curious and to listen.

There was at least one other GP at that time who was fascinated by health beliefs, he was also a genuine anthropologist. I met Cecil Helman on a couple of occasions in 1980 when he visited the Department of Experimental Psychology. He was South African by birth, but we shared the common bond of having both been ship's doctors some years earlier. Cecil died quite young but certainly left his mark. When I met him, he had been thinking of folk beliefs in medicine for a few years and even published an article on it as early as 1978. In 1981 he published the folk model we had discussed in the Oxford concourse. These are the questions people ask themselves when there is some perceived change in their health:

What has happened?
Why has it happened?
Why to me?
Why now?
What would happen if nothing were done about it?
What should I do about it?

At last, I had something I could understand myself and so teach to others. I was on a mission. Armed with seven consulting tasks, rules for running sensitive group discussions and a newly-realised enthusiasm for discovering what made the people who consulted me tick, I think I was soon insufferable. The Oxford groups I led were quite enthusiastic but, much like the curate's egg, only in parts. This was my obsession, not theirs. My partners treated me with a kind, slightly nervous, indulgence. My registrars probably benefited most, at least they could leave at the end of the year. The patients queued up, but they might have done anyway as we were a busy practice.

David Pendleton was now working with his wife Jenny in a management consultancy business they had set up, and was soon to move to Hong Kong. Theo and Peter were developing a five-day consulting course. I attended a few, as did David, but the other two really honed this course over nearly two decades and helped so many GPs to understand and improve their consulting. I wanted to push on, to take it further, but was unclear how.

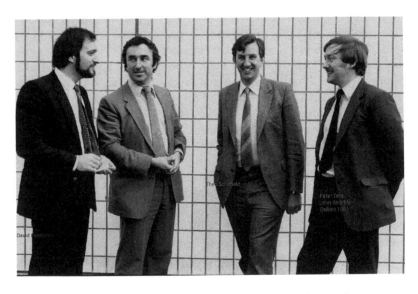

Outside the John Radcliffe in 1982. From left to right,
David Pendleton, Peter Havelock, Theo Schofield, Peter Tate.

I was admitted to the club of MRCGP Examiners in 1982. Theo Schofield was already one and Peter Havelock and I joined in the same intake. My oldest friend from university, Penrith GP Tony Reed, was a well-established examiner by this time. Joining the Panel was a considerable step up in professional development; the selection was daunting and by no means a shoe-in. The Panel was, and probably remains, a necessary thorn in the side of the greater organisation. It was passionately apolitical, pro-standard setting, with a corporate desire to raise the standards of the profession in the UK. At this time, the Panel wished to set the standard to join the RCGP, and this was deliberately to be set at an aspirational level rather, than as it has become, the basic level of entry into the profession. When I joined, the Chief Examiner was my old Professor of General Practice at Newcastle, John Walker, but he soon handed on the baton to Andrew Belton, a GP from Skipton, very near to my old school, Giggleswick.

Andrew Belton was a Yorkshireman, through and through. He was big, combative, wore studded leather jackets and cared, more than turned out to be good for him, about the educational attainments of young GPs. In 1984, during an oral viva examination session in Edinburgh he overheard his deputy and head of the oral examination, Andrew Marcus extolling the virtues of the new vegetarian restaurant, Henderson's (which is still there). This was too much for Andrew, the son of farming stock; he got together a group, including me, to go to Desperate Dan's (which is no longer there), the meat-eater's haven, where we gorged on huge skewers of steak, lamb, pork and sausage which probably raised the world's temperature by half a degree on its own. You can imagine the subsequent repartee.

In 1986, after a particularly frustrating diet of the examination, Andrew wrote a letter to The Times, stating baldly that, on the evidence of the MRCGP examination, young aspirational GPs did not appear to read very much, not of a medical nature anyway. The newspapers and medical magazines picked this up and there was a brief ripple in the pond.

At this time in 1986, I was coming to the end of my eight-year stint as an Oxford District Course organiser for vocational training. I had begun in 1978, met David Pendleton and it had changed my life. The Oxford region's advisor on general practice was John Hasler, a GP from Sonning Common, near Henley, who had risen quickly through the ranks with a combination of drive, intelligence, organisational skill and, fatally as it turned out, ambition. John was really the fifth author of *The Consultation* book and was David Pendleton's guiding star. He had his office at the top of the Old Radcliffe Observatory, beloved of Morse and Endeavour episodes. My office was at the bottom of the stairs where the corpses piled up. Soon we were evicted, to make way for the new Postgraduate Green College. I was given an office – more of a broom cupboard really – in the brand new Oxford hospital. The John Radcliffe Hospital was to be a significant influence on so many lives including my own. It was covered in gleaming white tiles and was affectionately, but sarcastically, known as The John.

One evening in late summer that year, a very influential group were having a private meeting in a corner of the RCGP College bar in Prince's Gate. The most important member of this cabal was Donald Irvine, an Ashington GP of boundless ambition, Regional Advisor for the Newcastle Region and recently retired Chair of the RCGP. I had sort of known Donald via my North East connections for several years. A year earlier, in 1985, he had attended the Examiner's Conference held at Glenridding, Ullswater; this was a tactical thing to do for a current chairman, but his method of transport was spectacularly over the top, arriving by helicopter. In his defence, he did strive hard to improve standards in general practice, and revolutionised the GMC several years later. He was knighted, but finally upset just too many people and fell, Icarus-like, from grace. Also present were Alastair Donald, a senior College grandee, a good man and past Chair of the RCGP, and John Lawson, who had also previously been Chair of Council. There are varied accounts of this overheard discussion, but the overall gist was that College Council could not allow such insubordination as Andrew Belton's, with his expression of semi-official, controversial and newsworthy opinions without official sanction. The reports suggest that the conversation called for his summary sacking from his position. The current Chair of RCGP Council at that time, John Hasler, was not part of this cabal but was informed later that, whatever misgivings he might have, this was the irrevocable decision and he would be supported in it. They lied.

The then-President, the affable and kindly Michael Drury, was handed the unenviable task, given Andrew's volatile persona, of informing him of this decision. The Examiners were thus forewarned of the coming storm. All hell broke loose, and for a week or two it looked like the Panel would resign en mass and the College would have no examination for the foreseeable future. At the Council meeting of 20th of September 1986, John Hasler read out a pre-prepared statement stating what a good man Andrew was and that, although he had not actually done anything wrong, he needed sacking for being too free with his opinions, or words to that effect. By the AGM (Annual General Meeting) of November that year John Hasler, looking round for those he thought his allies on the Council, found none and was forced to resign. I don't think he has ever been back to the College. Several senior examiners did resign, but enough stayed to keep it afloat. My friend, and John Hasler's deputy in Oxford, Northampton GP John Toby steadied the ship, and with ex-Chief Examiner John Walker (who incidentally was furious with fellow Newcastle man Donald Irvine, perceiving him as the real villain of the piece), rallied the examiners and remarkably produced a well-ordered October diet of the exam.

When I got back from America in February 1987, John Toby took me aside, walked me through the coming changes in examination structure and offered me the job of running the oral viva examination, a role newly given the title of Oral Convenor. The title of Chief Examiner was gone too; that became Convenor* of the Panel, answerable to a newly constituted Examination Board, itself answerable to the Council. The previous holder of my new job was of course Andrew Marcus, who had been one of those who resigned. He had been a good friend and mentor but never spoke to me again, perceiving that I had stolen his job. It really is a funny old world.

It was around this time that a new examiner joined the panel, one who was to make, and continues to make, a huge contribution to the development of doctor–patient communication, and not just in the UK. This was Roger Neighbour, newly returned from America with a head full of neuro-linguistic programming and sports coaching techniques. Roger, a GP in Kings Langley, came to the Examiners Conference in 1987 with a pile of the new books he had just published; *The Inner Consultation: How to Develop an Effective and Intuitive Consulting Style*'. This was uneasy for us Oxfordians, two Peters and Theo. We were a little proprietorial and here was a new boy jumping all over 'our turf'; a Cambridge man, with fresh, interesting and challenging ideas to boot. It took a while, but shared interest won over competition and a friendship developed that continues to this day. Roger was much better at linking tasks to skills than we had been, and his five tasks on one hand was a very clever idea. He called them the checkpoints in the consultation.

1. Connecting with the patient.
2. Summarising with the patient.
3. Handing over to the patient.
4. Safety netting (contingency plans and honest admission of uncertainties).
5. Housekeeping (taking care of yourself).

Over the years we climbed up the examinations ladder, both serving terms as Chief Examiner of the Panel, and Roger going on to be President of the College. Another examiner was David Haslam, a Huntingdon GP, also still a friend, who went on to be Chairman of the RCGP, the BMA

---

* The term Convenor was a mealy-mouthed cop out directly attributable to the Belton affair; I have reverted to Chief Examiner when describing this era for ease of understanding.

and NICE (National Institute for Health and Care Excellence). Dad would have hated him.

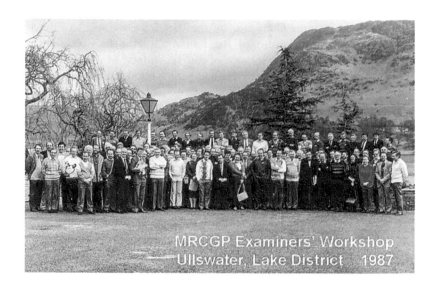

MRCGP Examiners' Workshop Ullswater, Lake District, 1987.

Running the oral examination was fun. The panel was 125-strong in the late 1980s, up to 200 by the millennium, and we ran four diets a year. Two in Prince's Gate, London and two in the Royal College of Physicians Library in Edinburgh. These doctors were banner-carriers for their chosen profession. Nothing staves off burnout better than regular exposure to enthusiasts, and I loved them all. I developed a strong friendship with the Examination Administrator Tom Dastur, unflappable, sartorially elegant, affable, un-sarcastic, diplomatic to a fault and by a long chalk the finest organiser I ever met. For a decade we travelled up to Edinburgh on the day before the examination to set out the tables and finalise last minute arrangements in the large, gloomy, forbidding and musty old, pillared Library. Our meanderings were scrutinised by severe, long-dead Scottish physicians whose portraits hung in the alcoves and emanated an unmistakable air of vague Presbyterian disapproval. We always ate the same meal at the same Chinese, had a similar conversation to last time, usually relating to the relentless ticking of the Library clock marking the passing of the years, had a quiet drink and went to bed early. Honestly, we were like a couple of old ... but you are not to say that anymore.

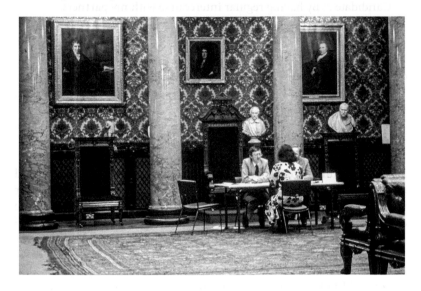

Royal College of Physicians, Edinburgh. Oral exam in progress, 1988.

Two examiners took on one candidate for a 30-minute oral; it was gladiatorial, intense, trained and, as far as we could make it, fair. The candidate had to do it twice. It was a real test. In the early 1990s Roger Neighbour and I were paired together. We were somewhat infamous at that time, and the candidates knew who we were; a young man on being introduced to us, looked heavenwards and said loudly 'Beam me up Scotty'. We did collect a few examples of funny responses between examiner and candidate; I give you just a few:

Examiner: What happens to bereaved people?
Candidate: They die more often.

Examiner: How can you keep your practice team's morale up?
Candidate: I would let the receptionists out at Christmas.

Examiner: How do you assess the depth of a patient's depression?
Candidate: You could ask them if they had committed suicide before?

Examiner: How do you avoid burnout?
Candidate 1: See more of my friend's wife, etc.
Candidate 2: By having regular intercourse with my partners.
Candidate 3: Go to Australia.

One of the cases I used to use in oral examinations was based on a true experience. It was intended to test the candidates' handling of maturity onset diabetes, and how they would cope in less than ideal circumstances. It was also meant to test racial undertones as the patient was a Romany lady, but the true story is far more interesting than my little oral crib cards that are in front of me as I write.

In the late 1970s a nervous young lady asked me to visit her mother. She didn't think there was too much wrong with her, but she just would not be able to come to the surgery, and she had not seen a doctor for years. She looked so pleading that I readily agreed and asked the address. There was a long hesitation, 'It would be better if I showed you'. So, she did. Down a long cart track on the edge of town there was a little clearing containing two small caravans. One was a beautiful Romany Caravan and the other a tatty, battered little grey one that a Morris Minor would have towed with ease. There were a couple of horses grazing. Disappointingly, I was led to the latter one. It was very small, blue with cigarette smoke and on this morning smelling strongly of bleach. A scrawny thin wisp of a man ghosted out and disappeared apparently into thin air.

'That's my Dad, he won't speak to you, scared of doctors'.

Across the tiny bunk table sat a small but bulky figure in full overcoat, lit by a small paraffin lantern in a way Caravaggio could not have improved on.

'This is my mum, Rose'.

As I started on the pleasantries of introduction Rose interrupted.

'My feet are numb, and my little toe is black. I think it might need to come off, but I am not going to hospital'.

In the MRCGP Oral Examination we used to teach examiners to set up difficult case scenarios, and then explore the candidate's options, the implications of those options and finally their choice, and why.

My brain was already rapidly scanning those options, but David P was sitting on my shoulder.

'What would you like me to do?'

And she told me. She assumed she had 'sugar' which had killed her mother too, and would need pills to bring it under control, no injections mind you. She would need help with her foot, and she couldn't come to the surgery because she smelt bad and it would upset the other patients. Skillfully rolling a small cigarette, she offered it to me, smiled at my refusal, lit it, took a drag and waited for my response. We negotiated an option, finally settling on her daughter bringing Rose to the surgery in the early morning before it was officially open. Here we could examine her properly, do the blood tests and get the district nurse involved. We did this, saved her toe and it was the start of a friendship. After that I visited her regularly, but not always in the same place; she was a true Romany but her travelling days were over. Rose made little concession to the sort of dietary and lifestyle advice the nurses and I tried to promulgate; she was happily but defiantly non-compliant, and I don't recall ever seeing her without a small, glowing tab hanging from her right lower lip.

'I am like this caravan, battered by life and I know I won't make old bones. We know you know … it's the second sight'.

I didn't think you needed the second sight to come to that conclusion, but you couldn't but recall the Indiana Jones line, 'It's not the age it's the mileage'. It transpired that Rose was of travelling fairground stock, and she had settled in Abingdon because of the Michaelmas Fair, originally a medieval hiring fair for rural farmworkers to find work in the local area. Over the years, more and more stalls and fairground rides were added to make it the longest street fair in Europe, running a mile down the length of the High Street from the marketplace and down Ock Street. For centuries, all the fairs in Oxfordshire and Berkshire had been in sequence, all slightly different to reflect their hometown. Rose had done them all since she was born and the Ock Street Fair was then, and remains, a big deal. In the early 1980s my wife and children would visit, and Rose would usually be in the marketplace with her collection of old children's boat swings; they would always get a free go, free sweets and a bit of attention. Right next door was the Gypsy Rose Lee fortune telling booth, who was one of Rose's close relatives, and one year she came out to meet me. We exchanged a few words and she took my hand, looked my left palm and into my eyes. 'You have been read before'. I was nonplussed; she led me into her tent.

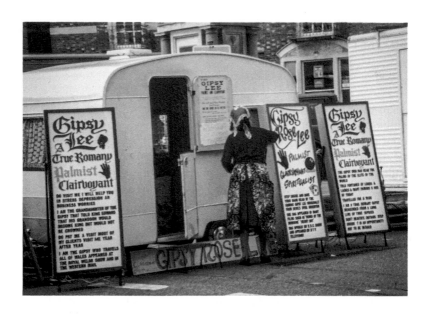

Ock Street Fair, 1985.

My father had looked after the fairground people of South Shields' medical needs, and as a 15-year-old I had my palm read as a treat. What she told me disquieted me considerably at the time and I shared the experience with my father but not my mother. I had asked a typical teenage question about how long my life line was, but the fortune teller had prevaricated, before eventually telling me that yes, I would live a reasonable time, but after 30 it might be more of a struggle. I would however, weather those adversities and have a reasonably successful life. For some reason this fairly bland and unspecific prognostication unsettled me and remained not too deep in my subconscious. To the extent that when I had my first pacemaker aged 30, I said to myself that the fortune teller had warned me.

This newer version was warm, thanked me for being kind to Rose, told me to look after my wife and told me something else, not for telling but that did transpire. My life has been full of scepticism, and I love Derren Brown's debunking of mediums and fake evangelists but sometimes, just sometimes, I wonder.

After nearly a decade Rose's own fortune telling came true, but while her death was expected, what a surprise was her funeral. She was, to use her own phrase, a Gipsy Queen and was treated in death such as she had never been treated in life. Here from her little, cold, bare-necessities caravan, with no running water or electricity, they took her ornate and opulently draped coffin to lead a procession, and what a procession! It was longer than the whole length of Ock Street. I stood by where she used to have her swings, and shed a tear as she passed regally by. She is the only royalty I have had the privilege of looking after.

In the late 1980s a group of us began to feel that the exam was not testing the parts of a doctor's armoury that really mattered – a young GP's consulting competence. Two competing philosophies emerged. Southampton GP Peter Burrows and Newbury GP Liz Bingham led the simulated surgery, or OSCE (objective structured clinical examination) group, using scripted actors in exam settings and marking the responses on an agreed proforma. If this was a competition it comes as no surprise to know they won, eventually. The other philosophy, led by me with Roger Neighbour, Birmingham GP Steve Field and Hull GP Peter Campion as close allies, thought that direct observation of actual performance was the best way to go. This was now possible, if clunky, using the VHS videotape format, which was cheap and available to all. Both groups made some early progress but then came against an apparently insurmountable barrier. Statistics.

At this time the Centre for Medical Education in Dundee, run by Professor Ron Harden, held the contract to oversee the statistical correctness of the various parts of the MRCGP examination. They were adamant that neither method would lend itself easily to a reproducible, valid, statistical analysis, but that the direct observation method was dead in the water. I asked our own brilliant, but alternative, exam psychometrician, Richard Wakeford, for his opinion; he thought they were wrong, but not entirely so. If we were to produce a new direct observation examination, a very different approach would be needed. Then a bit of complex politics occurred; Philip Tombleson, Chief Examiner of the Panel, urbane, charming and with a core of steel, took my side. I suspect there were other reasons too, but when the contract with Dundee came up for review, he vetoed it, and we put the job out to tender. A graduate in Medieval French from the University of Liverpool came to interview. He had subsequently specialised in statistical understanding and bamboozled us all at interview with small dissertations on skew and kurtosis and their effects on probability and distribution. He was also funny, amiable and destined to become another very good friend. He was John Foulkes, and it was late 1991.

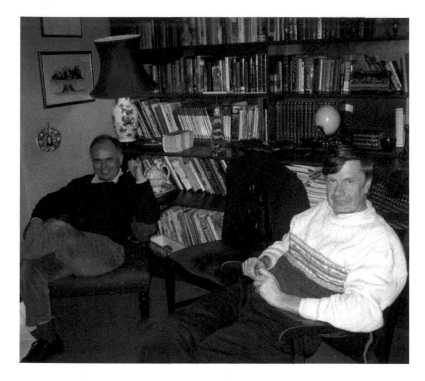

Roger Neighbour and John Foulkes.

REFERENCES

Kahneman D. 2011. *Thinking, Fast and Slow*. New York: Farrar, Straus and Giroux.

Helman CG. 1978. "Feed a cold, starve a fever" – Folk models of infection in an English suburban community, and their relation to medical treatment. *Cult Med Psychiatry*. 2, 107–137.

Neighbour R. 2005. *The Inner Consultation*, 2nd ed. Oxford: Radciffe Publishing.

6

The Video Examination

By 1991 the machinery of the RCGP was beginning to move in a helpful direction. Following the appointment of John Foulkes, the Examination Board appointed me to lead a group developing the concept of videotape assessment of consulting in practice. I had spent over a decade working towards this point and was raring to go. The MRCGP examination had long lacked a true 'clinical' component, unlike other medical examinations such as the Membership of the Royal College of Physicians and the Fellowship of the Royal College of Surgeons. What do GPs do? They consult with their patients. It was generally agreed that a consulting component was necessary. Obviously the OSCE approach had advantages in terms of reproducibility, but was greedy of manpower and space requirements. It was also not quite the real thing; a problem with most exams.

John Foulkes knew of Miller's Pyramid, a method of ranking clinical competence. As a framework, it distinguishes between knowledge at the lower levels and action in the higher levels. It argued that to truly know whether candidates are achieving what the RCGP want them to achieve, they should be assessed in the setting that we expect them to work, in the surgery. The most accepted definition of competence is that of a latent state of potentiality, or, in plainer English, it is that which a doctor knows and can utilise. This contrasts with performance, which relates to the reality of day-to-day work; in other words what doctors actually do in their surgeries.

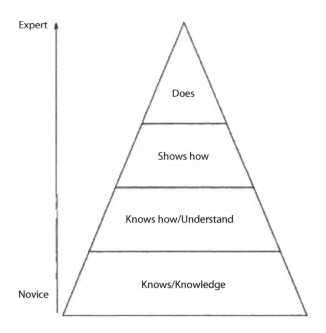

Miller's Pyramid. (Source: Miller GE. The assessment of clinical skills/competence/performance. *Acad Med* 1990;65(suppl):S63–67. PubMedWeb of ScienceGoogle Scholar.)

In this model the highest level is the 'does' level; in other words, how the doctor actually performs in the consulting room. To assess at this level requires some form of direct observation, sitting in, a one-way screen, a simulated patient unknown to the doctor in a real setting, or most commonly at this time, a video recording of doctor–patient encounters. The 'shows how' level is usually assessed by role-play, OSCEs and consulting simulations; these methodologies are inherently less authentic because they involve artificial and arranged clinical scenarios, but they are powerful, formative tools. There is a difficulty with such methods when used for regulatory purposes because of the leap of faith required to be convinced that competence demonstrated by such assessments actually translates into real performance.

Further down the pyramid the 'knows how' level is often assessed by face-to-face tutorials in formative assessments, and by oral examinations in regulative assessments. Results from the MRCGP examination had clearly demonstrated that 'knows how' consulting knowledge, as expressed by candidates in the oral examination, demonstrated knowledge of patient-centred consulting at a level of around 85% of candidates; it was actually demonstrated by candidates in their submitted videotape in about 10% of candidates.

The 'knows' level is usually assessed for formative and research purposes by questionnaire and rating scales, and for regulative purposes with written examinations. A brief glance at the pyramid makes it unsurprising that results from written examinations correlate poorly with actual performance. The simple rule is that the greater the veracity required of the assessment instrument, the higher up the pyramid you have to go. Some would argue that the word veracity could be substituted with validity. For the MRCGP we were interested in what candidates can do, which then, with a bit of wishful thinking, we hoped they might do in practice.

We felt direct observation of real consultations was more valid than simulation; whether we could make it reliable was the real issue. To tell the truth, I was only peripherally interested in reliability, to the extent that what mattered to me was the educational stimulus given by the new examination to produce more effective doctors in the UK. Reliability was a hurdle to jump, and it was a high one. Dundee had said it was impossible.

There is a beguilingly simple formula that can be used to quantify the usefulness of an assessment tool. Utility of assessment tool = Validity × Reliability × Feasibility × Acceptability × Educational impact. If there are serious deficiencies in any of the five areas listed, then the usefulness of the tool must be questioned.

Regulatory assessments are designed to discriminate between candidates; this is the purpose of the assessment. A measure designed to assess minimal competence, at say the 95% acceptance level, is going to be a different animal from that which seeks to measure optimal competence at a particular stage of apprenticeship, say allowing 70% to progress through. A final, later career measure such as Fellowship might reasonably anticipate a 50% initial pass rate.

VALIDITY

Validity is a complex issue. The arguments can get very academic and are concerned with two fundamental questions; the extent to which an assessment method actually measures what it is designed to measure, and what are the relationships between the variable measured and the other variables. John Foulkes was fundamental to helping us think through the main areas of validity. For those who are interested, I have included a description of the issues around validity that we had to deal with in the Appendix.

RELIABILITY

Then there was reliability, on the face of it a simpler concept. Reliability is the extent to which one can rely on the result of an assessment to accurately measure the item to be assessed. For example, single measurements of blood pressure will vary because of fluctuations in the blood pressure itself, subject variation, measurement errors in the machine used to take the pressure and differences between the same observers at different times (intra-observer variation) or between different observers (inter-observer variation). Reliability can be increased by steps such as repeated measures, increasing the precision of the criteria for the assessment, multiple observers and assessor training. If an assessment rating scale has multiple items, it is possible to establish the correlation between the scores for each item. Low levels of correlation would suggest that the scores might vary randomly; high levels of correlation mean that some of the items may be redundant. Reliability measurements are bedevilled by a bewildering variety of statistical methodologies; two of the most important are Cronbach's alpha and kappa. The first is a measure of the internal consistency of the tool, with figures above 0.8 being acceptable for regulatory instruments. The second is a measure of inter-rater reliability and is the hardest measure to achieve acceptable levels.

Human communication is complex; it is often the subtleties that make the difference. Achieving good reliability while simultaneously measuring what really matters is not an easy task; many assessments fall at this hurdle. Reliability is most important for regulatory assessment; careers are on the line. In our case, an important element of reliability is the repeatability of the instrument, so that it generates similar results from cohort to cohort. Generalisability is a significant, related concept to reliability, affecting decisions such as how many consultations need to be watched to form a reliable judgement. There are two issues here. The first is whether the performance observed on a single occasion is representative of usual performance; the good or bad day phenomenon. The second is the extent to which one can safely generalise performance in one area to other areas. The evidence is that some doctors may have some skills but not others, and can handle some situations better than others. A reliable assessment therefore depends on an adequate sample, covering a range of skills and situations.

FEASIBILITY

Then the next part of that deceptively simple little formula, feasibility. This was a big one. Regulatory and research assessments are most affected by this consideration. For example, a 20-station simulation may have high reliability but the logistics of running such an examination for say, 2,000 candidates a year, are massive. Without an efficient major organisation behind it, such a regulatory methodology becomes unfeasible. A similar project on a local basis for much smaller numbers may be quite do-able. We were thinking of 2,000 videotapes a year being made, sent for examination, watched by trained assessors and ending up with accurately collated and defensible results.

ACCEPTABILITY

For assessments to be effective, they must be acceptable to all involved; the assessed, the assessors and our patients. This was not easy to achieve. Assessing consulting performance, and so inferring the degree of competence, is an emotive issue. No doctor wishes to be found wanting in this central area of his or her being. This perceived emotional threat is one reason for the oft-stated dislike of both formative and regulative assessments. Those being assessed had to be convinced of the merits of the method, before they were be prepared to subject themselves to it. Of course, if the assessment was imposed but seen as flawed by many, this would generate considerable resentment, and a climate not conducive to improving consulting. This meant that both examiners and candidates had to be involved, feel committed to the process and derive educational benefits from it, else why do it?

EDUCATIONAL IMPACT

A good-quality regulatory assessment will influence the learners' and teachers' agendas for the better, at any stage in the medical voyage. The corollary is regrettably also true; a poor assessment will set back consulting development. It remains a challenge for all who care about the importance of good communication between doctor and patient, that the educational impact of any assessment methodology should be a positive one. If the influence is malign in any way, such as demotivating, deskilling or perhaps too divisive, then the assessment must be looked at, and if modification is unhelpful, it should be rejected.

John Foulkes thought he saw a way forward through this. He began exploring the NVQ (National Vocational Qualification) methodology. This is a work-based qualification which recognises the skills and knowledge a person needs to do a job. The candidate needs to demonstrate and prove their competency in their chosen role or career path. This, to our knowledge, was the first time such a structure was to be used in complex medical examinations. What we now had to do was produce a set of competencies that the panel of examiners could agree on. Since standards are an expression of a social construct, it is not possible to determine whether a particular standard is 'correct' or valid in the classic scientific sense (Kane, 1994). Instead, it was important to develop a body of procedural evidence and outcomes data that addressed the issue of credibility. Specifically, standards needed to be set by the right number and kind of standard-setters, the method we used to set them would need to meet certain criteria, and the outcomes of applying these standards should be reasonable (Norcini and Shea, 1997).

We started with our seven consulting tasks and went from there. With the help of Roger Neighbour, David Haslam and Lesley Southgate, we had soon produced five core competencies, or tasks.

1. Discover the reasons for a patient's attendance.
2. Define the clinical problems.
3. Address the patient's problems.
4. Explain the problems to the patient.
5. Make effective use of the consultation.

Very soon we had several sub-competencies required to complete the five tasks; 21 competencies in all. The examiners were very helpful and long-suffering, and began sending us videotapes of themselves consulting in their surgeries that we then tested the new methodology on. This was enlightening, without necessarily being helpful. Some were very competent, some were not (we lied about this in the paper we published). We became aware that we were walking on eggshells; what we were developing was an end-point assessment, there was no feedback built in at that stage. As an established doctor, to fail such an examination might well be devastating, a repudiation of one's whole career. There were no good points first here. A small worm of doubt crawled into my brain; could we do more harm than good? I kept telling John that we had a tiger by the tail; he said this was not helpful. Meanwhile, the GMC put up a lot of obstacles regarding patient confidentiality, and it took all of the new Chief Examiner Professor Lesley Southgate's soothing and political skills, which she had in abundance; I did not, politics is not a strength. We stuttered along for a year or two until finally getting the go ahead in 1993. By now, Steve Field and Peter Campion had joined the group, and David Haslam had gone off to chair the Examination Board. It was then that I had one of those rare phone calls that changes lives.

This call was from an old patient and friend who worked in medical publishing, and had been with Blackwells in Oxford for several years. He had some news for me, could I meet him at The George and Dragon in Sutton Courtney in half an hour? It was a lovely, late winter day in early 1993. I walked across the Thames from Culham, and there was Andrew

Bax waiting for me, looking a little nervous. Over a couple of beers he told me he was setting up his own publishing company, Radcliffe Medical Press, he had a couple of authors lined up, particularly Michael Drury with *The Medical Receptionist's Handbook*, but he needed something up-to-date for doctors, on communication preferably, as he thought that would be a good start. It took a while for the penny to drop as I suggested a couple of names and he shook his head. 'You want me to write it?' He grinned and nodded. 'Can you call it *The Doctor's Communication Handbook*, and oh yes, can I have it by Tuesday as there is a bit of a hurry with cash flow and all that'. So, there it was. Luckily it was all in my head. My then registrar was Mark Mayall, who was already and remains a good friend, so I sat down with my Amstrad computer and its early word-processing programme Locoscript, and imagined talking to Mark about studying the consultation. It was a chance to write a handbook that would guide candidates through the new examination. It just flowed out onto the page; I don't remember if I made Tuesday, but it wasn't far off. It actually took nearly a year to be published. As I write this, 25 years later, the eighth edition has recently been published, which is hard to believe.

My favourite review by a country mile was Roger's, written in November 1993:

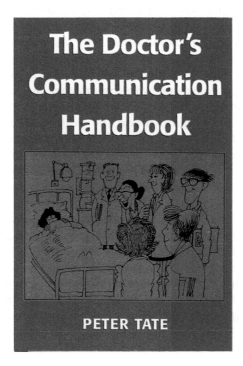

'You get the impression that, to some authors, writing about general practice feels much the same as truffle-hunting must do to the pig. Not an ordinary pig, you understand, such as is happy in muck. A pig with attitude. A pig with aspirations. A pig in the wrinkle of whose brow hauteur hopes to pass for breeding. A pig who although reduced to grubbing for a living goes home at night to a sty crammed with alabaster busts of the late Sir Porker and the thirteenth Baron Saddleback. A pig, in short, who can just about cope with getting its feet dirty as long as it sports a dab of something by Chanel behind the ears to waft to the workaday world a faintly protesting, "Oh that it should come to this"'.

And again, you get the impression that, to some casual observers, general practice must appear virtually indistinguishable from golf. The skilled practitioner of both activities knows this to be no sneer but actually a rather sharp insight. The essence of both is the same compulsive stalking of something small, wilful, immune to threat and entreaty, but desperately and disproportionately important; the same frustration of no sooner lighting on one option – one club, one line to the hole – than having seven others suggest themselves; the same ungainly contortions of mortal flesh attempting to approximate itself to the elegant ideals of the demigods; and above all the same recurring crushing awareness that the technical difficulties are as moonlight unto sunlight compared with the internal invisible demonic battle against doubt and self-criticism.

And so, to my good friend the golf-renouncing truffle-eschewing Peter Tate, formerly one-third of the Pendletonian 'et al.' and now sole author of The Doctor's Communication Handbook, I send a copy of Dorothy Parker's telegram to her puerperal chum – 'Congratulations. We all knew you had it in you'.

Bravo Pete. The loin-fruit manages to be both beautiful and the spitting image of its Dad. I've always thought single-author books had more oomph, and this one is an uninhibited paean of good communication by someone who reckons talking with patients to be one of the performing arts and not an academic discipline. I'm sure it wasn't written this way (it was!); but you'd think Peter had taken his favourite medical student, his favourite trainee and his favourite god-child and entertained them over dinner and long into the night with the dictaphone switched on. As a result, his book has a fluency and an immediacy that more than compensate for the occasional gung-ho moment, e.g. 'The GP's primary duty is to protect patients from hospital medicine'.

There are some lovely cameos breathing life into yes – Ideas, Concerns and Expectations, health beliefs and a few new friends such as the 'locus of control'. The classic Pendleton analysis is still here, with its seven tasks recast into a subdivided five. Pete's chapter on consultation strategies and skills is full of good ideas, several of them his own (I love that line): 'Closing the notes can signal the end of the consultation. Wearing a dinner jacket tends to speed patients up a bit but cannot be used too often. Taking the chair away is a last resort'.

Quite a few sacred cows lie bleeding after Tate has motored by. Here he is on 'the current craze for giving lifestyle advice. To come to your doctor with a cold and be told to stop smoking, lose weight, have your cervix smeared, your breasts examined and your cholesterol measured, and, to boot, that you can't have any cough mixture prescribed for you, may to a large section of the community be profoundly unsatisfying. However, the profession as a whole by a majority verdict would probably consider this good practice'. Or, on people who believe themselves to be in charge of their own health destiny, and who 'will not have an aluminium pot in the house for fear of Alzheimer's and who are to be found sweating in health food shops rummaging for the elixir of life having just run five miles to get there. (These people) tend to get very cross if they do get ill. To spend 20 years abstaining from the good things in life to keep one's cholesterol below five and then still have a coronary at 55 makes for a very unhappy and disillusioned human being.' Or, on the totally patient-centred doctor, 'probably a dangerous creature. Patients ... don't expect a laid-back hippie to let them do all the talking, planning and managing for themselves'. That's the Peter Tate I know and love, the iconoclastic epicure with the external locus of control who 'reckons in this life God gives you a certain number of heartbeats and I'm buggered if I'm wasting any of mine running round in bloody circles on wet Sunday mornings!'

> *Though you mightn't think it from the title, one of the best bits is the chapter on Informed Consent and other ethical issues. The following one is also excellent, on special problems like breaking bad news and dealing with angry or somatising patients. The abiding impression is of a wise and compassionate doctor with affection bordering on love for the work he does and the people he cares for, and who longs to have his pupils appreciate the same warmth and closeness. The book is engaging and does indeed engage; and an engaged reader is more than half wedded to the author's passion. Again, bravo'.*

It was remarkably well received, and in 1995 was awarded a Highly Commended Certificate in the BMA awards; I mention this because it was given exactly same award 20 years later in 2015, for the seventh edition.

Around this time, Roger and I were invited to a French, Quebec and English conference on the latest developments in doctor–patient communication. It was to be in Nice, which sounded nice. I was to speak on the new video examination, and Roger was to present some of his thoughts from his books. The fly in the ointment was that the conference would be in French, but we were promised most would be English speakers. Roger's linguistic education was far superior to mine; he translated my talk for me and promised to help with questions.

On the first night things did not go well. I was surrounded by garrulous French doctors who spoke not a word of English to me, and did not help with my stumbling Englishman-abroad attempts at conversation. The next day, with some trepidation, I gave my French speech. There is a bit of the thespian within me, and I delivered it with as much panache and best Giggleswick School French accent as I could muster. It was well received, with much applause, followed by questions. A collapse of the stout party ensued, Roger was gone and my French was not up to it, but a friendly Quebecois helped out. That evening everyone talked to me in English. I had passed some sort of test; the French are like that. One evening we went to a café in town, drank too much and sang a lot of pretty rude songs, mainly about Germans, which improved my language skills immeasurably.

Some years later *The Doctor's Communication Handbook* was translated into French *'Soigner (aussi) sa communication'* and in 2006 was awarded Le Prix Prescrire, one of France's top medical literary awards. The presentation was in Paris, but I could not attend, and my French was no better.

Meanwhile, back at the ranch as they say, in 1995, we carried on with the examination development. We were developing a workbook for candidates, and trying to work out how many consultations we needed to review to produce a valid and reliable assessment. We settled on marking seven chosen by the candidate, as the best compromise between range and practicality. By now the philosophy of the exam was clear in our heads. We would tell the candidates what competences they had to demonstrate, give them detailed advice on these competencies and ask them to submit seven consultations of them doing what was required.

The workbook explained to candidates that

This assessment is based on the concept of competency, meaning that combination of knowledge, skills and attitudes which, when applied to a particular situation, leads to a given outcome… consulting skill competences have been specified that, for example, require the candidate to demonstrate the ability to discover the reasons for a patient's attendance, by eliciting their symptoms, which includes two competences: encouraging the patient to 'spill the beans', and not ignoring cues. We do not specify how the patient is encouraged to give their account of their symptoms: this may be by open questions, by appropriate use of silence, or some other way. Nor do we need to specify how the cues are responded to. We do expect that at least some bits of unsolicited information are picked up by the doctor. Thus, a competence is a complex skill, the possession of which is demonstrated by achieving the relevant performance criterion. Possession of the competence does not imply that the doctor uses it all the time. However, unless the candidate demonstrates the competence in action, we cannot assume they possess it. The Membership examination/MAP therefore looks for what you as a candidate can do.

The time scale for collecting these videoed consultations would be approximately seven to eleven months. We realised that it took time to produce a video tape of seven consultations that demonstrated the competencies required. Most registrars probably needed to record at least five consultations for every one they submitted. Say 35–40 over a year, or less than one a week. We knew most trainers agreed that there should be some review of consulting at least once a month, so, say the candidate submitted their tape in the eighth month, thcy would have had at least seven sessions, watching say four or five a time.

There were, however, a number of trainers and registrars who objected to this process, feeling the time could be better spent elsewhere, and that the preparation for the MRCGP somehow got in the way of training. This group advocated a simulation examination, avoiding the perceived tedious and unhelpful preparation. Looking back, who was right? Did assessment drive learning, and if it did, was it not reasonable to expect that a serious postgraduate examination needs practice and demonstrable expertise in the workplace to pass? When the MRCGP examination introduced a critical reading paper in the late 1980s it was done to stimulate reading in registrars, and research subsequently showed it had the desired effect, except on poor Andrew Belton. The video examination was introduced to improve consulting. Even those who advocated a simple end-point, simulated examination must concede that to become a proficient consulter requires practice, intelligent feedback and more practice. Good consulting is truly skilful, like playing the piano well, and not many can do that without regular practice and tuition. General practice is currently the last refuge of the true generalist, and the major skill of the generalist is to really communicate and, to use Roger Neighbour's check point, 'connect' with our patients. This skill is not God-given, most doctors do not possess it at the beginning of training, or even at the end, and the assessments designed to measure this skill must, I still believe, encourage regular, rigorous performance review.

The medical press began taking an interest, and the article below from 1995, published in *Doctor Magazine,* highlights some of the profession's perceptions of this new examination, rightly or wrongly.

The very idea of amateur videos conjures up visions of Jeremy Beadle. Few people feel the dreaded camcorder does them any justice. And there cannot be many professionals who relish the thought of shots being used as part of an important exam or assessment.

But camcorder-shy GP trainees may have to learn to live with their small-screen images. Video assessment is almost an inevitability for future entrants to general practice and for those seeking membership of the GPs' royal college.

...The argument is that clinical knowledge alone does not make an effective GP – the consultation is the crux of successful general practice. Without good communication skills, doctors can all too easily miss the diagnostic clues presented by their patients. This fundamental aspect of the

trainee's ability is assessed by the trainer alone. But to meet the demands of the new legislation, the profession will have to come up with a more objective test. And the front runner is in-surgery video. The technique is also a hot favourite at the RCGP, where it is highly likely to be adopted as part of the membership exam.

...Now that the ethical niceties have been sorted out the trial is due to start this spring. GP Dr Peter Tate, of Abingdon, Oxfordshire – Convenor of the consulting skills component of the MRCGP – explains why the college is taking so much interest in video assessment.

'The MRCGP exam does not directly assess what GPs do – it assesses what they say they would do' he says. 'That is why I was asked, three or four years ago, to look to develop a method for directly assessing GPs' consulting skills. One of the obvious ways was to use videotape – it's cheap, it's familiar to everyone and it's been in use in vocational training for the past ten years or so'.

...Candidates examined during the pilot will be asked to video a wide range of consultations, following a carefully drawn-up patient-consent protocol, and submit the best examples for assessment. They will be required to include specific types of consultation – such as paediatric, geriatric and chronic disease management. And the video will be accompanied by a detailed workbook noting the GP's thoughts, feelings and ideas during each consultation. The aim is to establish clinical competence, according to a definition compiled by an RCGP working group.

...Dr Tate says an expanded version of this definition will be made clear to all candidates before the examination. He insists that the college is not trying to catch candidates out. The examiners will not be looking for expert handling of complex cases. The intention is to ensure GPs are able to fulfil the fundamental aims of the general practice consultation. And he hopes most candidates will already be familiar with, and unalarmed by, the idea of videoed consultations by the time the exam is established.

But there is a world of difference between watching a recording with a well-known trainer and sending videos to be inspected by strangers. There are bound to be fears that shy trainees and MRCGP candidates will be at a *disadvantage compared with more extrovert doctors. Some candidates might even seek training on performing for the camera.*

Dr Tate is adamant no special training will be needed. He says all doctors need is to get used to using video during consultations. 'If we are getting doctors that frightened, there is something wrong with the assessment method. All we want to do is film doctors working, not performing for the camera'.

Getting the Exam Panel to agree on the necessary performance criteria was no easy task, and our piloting experiences were salutary, and a little depressing at the same time. The young registrars who were volunteering for the pilots turned out to be not as proficient as hoped when measured against the 21 performance criteria; we had a frightening 80% fail rate. John Foulkes and I did several road shows in various parts of the country, and discovered that we both loved dreadful cowboy songs and old radio detective mysteries, particularly Ian Carmichael's *Lord Peter Wimsey*. We also found that the methodology was understood, and cautiously welcomed, by the training community. Nervously, we went back to the panel and recruited a further 40 experienced examiners who seemed keen. We did better this time. Even when using the full criteria, the examiners passed, most very easily. Our piloting showed marked improvements too, as the training community got to grips with the new assessment, but there was still a significant, but small, subsection of trainers who did worse (sometimes much worse) than their trainees. At last we had an instrument that seemed to differentiate the novice from the competent expert, most of the time. Now we needed to calibrate it.

We used a modified Delphi technique on the 130-strong Panel of Examiners, which is a fancy, academic way of saying that we asked them which performance criteria were most important; in other words, to rank them. If over 50% of the panel agreed, the criteria became mandatory. Initially the list was very doctor-centred (I was back to my Byrne & Long days), but the development did not stop there as, after all, the real point of the exercise was to increase patient-centredness in UK general practice consultations. We ploughed on, a couple of years went by, we told the Panel that this basic list was just that, basic, and was setting the exam at the level of minimal competence what they really wanted? After the second Delphi we climbed up to 11 mandatory criteria.

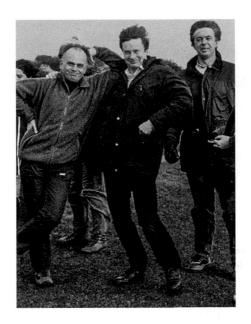

Roger, John and David Hallam, 1984.

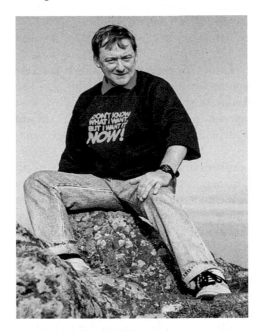

Me, 1993.

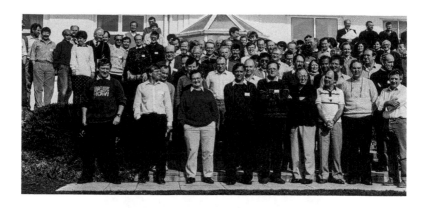

Panel of Examiners, 1993.

The Mandatory Performance Criteria to be demonstrated for Examinations in 1996 and 1997:

1. The doctor encourages the patient's contribution at appropriate points in the consultation.
2. The doctor responds to cues.
3. The doctor elicits appropriate details to place the complaint(s) in a social and psychological context.
4. The doctor obtains sufficient information for no serious condition to be missed.
5. The doctor chooses an examination which is likely to confirm or disprove hypotheses which could reasonably have been formed OR is designed to address a patient's concern.
6. The doctor appears to make a clinically appropriate working diagnosis.
7. The doctor explains the diagnosis, management and effects of treatment.
8. The doctor explains in language appropriate to the patient.
9. The doctor's management plan is appropriate for the working diagnosis, reflecting a good understanding of modern accepted medical practice.
10. The doctor shares management options with the patient.
11. The doctor's prescribing behaviour is appropriate.

The first full-scale diet of this video examination was in 1996. That it worked as well as it did was primarily down to organisation. Tom Dastur, exam organiser extraordinaire, deserves the credit, served ably by his deputy Sandra McKenzie. We used Radcliffe House, part of the Coventry Campus of the University of Warwick. All rooms needed up-to-date video recorders, and the system of sequential marking made 3D chess look like child's play.

But we did it, the examiners were reasonably happy, and knew a lot more about the state of modern general practice consulting at the end of it.

To be an effective educational tool, which was what we wished, the methodology had to allow constructive feedback to the candidate in the event of a failure, within this component of the examination. This was in the spirit of the examination being an integral part of the educational process. The use of specific performance criteria allowed this; candidates were informed about which performance criteria they failed to provide evidence of competence against. This explicit information enabled such candidates to concentrate on those areas of performance highlighted by the assessment, and to resubmit further evidence, we hoped with increased confidence.

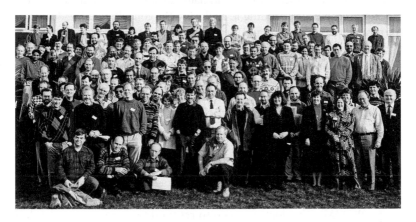

The Panel of Examiners, 1997.

In 1998 the MRCGP examination adopted a modular format. The videotaped consulting skills assessment became one of the four new modules. The requirements of the reorganised examination meant that the video assessment needed to be able to award a 'merit' pass for outstanding candidates, as well as making pass or fail decisions. To achieve this end, all 100 trained video examiners took part in a third modified Delphi technique to ascertain if there were any performance criteria that should become mandatory, and which criteria should be demonstrated in order to be awarded a merit. This process resulted in the development of three new merit criteria:

1. The doctor takes the patient's health understanding into account.
2. The doctor explains to the patient, utilising some or all of the patient's elicited beliefs.
3. The doctor tries to confirm the patient's understanding.

We began giving clearer examples of the sorts of behaviours we were looking for, and some of the behaviours that we did not want to see:

'Let's leave your headaches and talk about your cholesterol'.
'Here's a tissue, now when is your next mammogram?'
'You're here for your BP check, up with the sleeve...'
'I think smoking is more important to discuss than your legs, don't you...?'

A doctor from Hong Kong, desperate to impress the examiners with his patient-centredness, gave every patient a teddy bear at the end of each consultation. In another video, a candidate had obviously not looked through the submission before sending it, as during the consultation the doctor left the room to get a urine pot, and the young man spotted the video, smiled and then gave a full-blooded V sign. Most examiners knew how he felt.

By 2005, the performance criteria, after several iterations and additions looked like this; a thoroughly comprehensive and detailed dissection of the consultation, and the performance criteria (PC) needing to be demonstrated to show competence (P), and merit level (M).

Discover the reasons for the patient's attendance:

a. Elicit an account of the symptom(s):
   i. PC1 (P): The doctor is seen to encourage the patient's contribution at appropriate points in the consultation.
   ii. PC2 (M): The doctor is seen to respond to signals (cues) that lead to a deeper understanding of the problem.
b. Obtain relevant items of social and occupational circumstances:
   i. PC3 (P): The doctor uses appropriate psychological and social information to place the complaint(s) in context.
c. Explore the patient's health understanding:
   i. PC4 (P): The doctor explores the patient's health understanding.

Define the clinical problem(s):

a. Obtain additional information about the symptoms, and other details of medical history:
   i. PC5 (P): The doctor obtains sufficient information to include or exclude likely relevant significant conditions.
b. Assess the patient by appropriate physical and mental examination:
   i. PC6 (P): The physical/mental examination chosen is likely to confirm or disprove hypotheses that could reasonably have been formed OR is designed to address a patient's concern.

c. Make a working diagnosis:
    i. PC7 (P): The doctor appears to make a clinically appropriate working diagnosis.

Explain the problem(s) to the patient:

a. Share the findings with the patient:
    i. PC8 (P): The doctor explains the problem or diagnosis in appropriate language.
    ii. PC9 (M): The doctor's explanation incorporates some or all of the patient's health beliefs.
b. Ensure that the explanation is understood and accepted by the patient:
    i. PC10 (M): The doctor specifically seeks to confirm the patient's understanding of the diagnosis.

Address the patient's problem(s):

a. Choose an appropriate form of management:
    i. PC11 (P): The management plan (including any prescription) is appropriate for the working diagnosis, reflecting a good understanding of modern accepted medical practice.
b. Involve the patient in the management plan:
    i. PC12 (P): The patient is given the opportunity to be involved in significant management decisions.

Make effective use of the consultation:

a. Make effective use of resources:
    i. PC13 (M): In prescribing the doctor takes steps to enhance concordance, by exploring and responding to the patient's understanding of the treatment.
    ii. PC14 (P): The doctor specifies the conditions and interval for follow up or review.

Here are the descriptions we gave for the merit criteria:

1. PC2 (M): The doctor is seen to respond to signals (cues) that lead to a deeper understanding of the problem:
    Responding to cues is seen as a key component of 'active listening'. As you listen to the patient's story, you are sensitive both to what they say, how they say it and sometimes what they don't say. You are watching their face, and their 'body language', and use this

competency to explore areas which they might otherwise have passed over. You may also find cues in the records. There is no simple formula, but 'you said earlier….., what did you mean by that?' is an example of how this might be done. Similarly, 'I note that you haven't been to the doctor for over 10 years' might enable the patient to explain more fully what they were worried about. This PC is only demonstrated when as a result of the doctor's response to the cue, some additional information is elicited, leading to a 'deeper understanding of the problem'.

2. PC9 (M): The doctor's explanation incorporates some or all of the patient's health beliefs:

The beliefs to which this refers might or might not have been explicitly elicited, but have emerged during the consultation. This PC requires that the doctor incorporates one or more of the patient's ideas (about the nature or cause of their problem) into their explanation.

3. PC10 (M): The doctor specifically seeks to confirm the patient's understanding of the diagnosis:

Although currently a 'merit' criterion, checking that your explanation has been understood should be routine, except perhaps where the situation is obvious, or where there has been no new diagnosis, although even here, there is a place for checking the patient's understanding of even pre-existing conditions. It requires more than a cursory 'is that clear?' to which the answer is usually 'Yes doctor'. Better 'I don't know whether that makes sense, is there anything you want to ask me?', or 'how would you explain your condition to someone else?'

4. PC13 (M): In prescribing the doctor takes steps to enhance concordance, by exploring and responding to the patient's understanding of the treatment:

This new merit PC is based on the recent evidence that most patients do not adequately understand their treatment, nor take it as intended. There are two elements: exploring the patient's understanding of the treatment (analogous to PC 10, which explores their understanding of the diagnosis), plus a reactive explanation of the treatment in the light of this.

What the RCGP now possessed was the biggest consulting laboratory in the world. So, what did we learn?

REFERENCES

Byrne P & Long B. 1976. *Doctors Talking to Patients*. London: Royal College of General Practitioners Publications.

Kane M. 1994. Validating the performance standards associated with passing scores. *Review of Educational Research*, 64(3), 425–461.

Miller GE. 1990. The assessment of clinical skills/competence/performance. *Academic Medicine*, 65(suppl), S63–567.

Norcini JJ & and Shea JA. 1997. The credibility and comparability of standards. *Applied Measurement in Education*, 10(1), 39–59.

7

Other Foreign Adventures

Before we move on, a brief hiatus. It was in 1988, after my American experience, that an old friend approached me with a proposition. Peter Pritchard was a pioneering GP in the new village of Berinsfield, quite close to both Abingdon and Oxford. He was very active in local medical and social affairs, and his particular enthusiasm was patient participation in healthcare. Our consultation work was pivotal to a lot of his thinking. He had set up an Oxford educational collaboration, the UK Nordic Medical Educational Trust, along with the then Professor of General Practice in Oxford, Godfrey Fowler, whose wife was Scandinavian, and leading Oxford academic GP Martin Lawrence, all good friends.

The proposition was to teach the consulting tasks to groups of Swedish GPs who would be housed in one of the Oxford colleges out of term time, usually Pembroke. Initially this was sporadic, over a period of years, but it did help to develop the teaching technique of dividing groups into three or four, role-playing or discussing consultation techniques in Swedish, followed by larger group debriefing sessions in their second language English, with a bit of translation from the better English speakers.

In 1992 this occasional activity became extremely lucrative, due to the appearance of a new stomach medicine. The Swedish drug firm Hässle, a subsidiary of Astra, had developed Lansoprazole, a new proton-pump inhibitor, known in the UK as Losec (Prevacid in the USA). Hässle considerably increased their sponsorship of our courses, and as a result my remuneration increased considerably and the work became a lot more frequent. Throughout much of the 1990s I travelled to Sweden to run the same workshops there. My ironic sense of humour was in tune with the Scandinavian vibes, probably because my grandfather was Norwegian. I always began lectures by apologising in Swedish '*Jag talar inte svenska*' (I don't speak Swedish) and telling them that I was Al (as in Pendleton et al.), but I had sold my soul to a drug firm, although I never actually promoted the drug myself. I could work up some fake regret to fit in with modern feelings, but like to convince myself that over the years I did more good than harm. Ben Goldacre would not approve.

I have many jumbled memories of my Swedish trips, always accompanied by Hässle's Senior Director, Goran Aman. One is of the time we were being driven to Loka Brunn by an extremely well-oiled lady GP, who was clinging to the steering wheel and, with her face as close as she could get to the windscreen, navigating up the twisty and foggy mountain road, repeating again and again, 'I hope there no elk, I hope there no elk'. The place began as a health spa for Swedish royalty, but is now a posh conference centre for the hoi polloi. I soon found myself, stark naked, in the sauna next to an attractive lady Professor of Infectious Diseases, who was berating me on the UK deficiencies in Chlamydia screening. Agony would not adequately describe the feelings induced, but they would describe the feelings of the organiser of the whole event, who developed acute appendicitis in the middle of the night.

Another time I flew up to Örebro, then overshadowed by a huge ski jump which I think is now demolished. I was greeted warmly and taken off to a colleague's dacha on the coast. There was a lot of grinning and nervous shuffling when lunch was mentioned; something was afoot. 'Did I like herring?' With my South Shields heritage, how could I not. There was more nervous laughter, and a lady GP squeezed my hand as if in sympathy. Then there was the smell; what a smell, it haunts me still. What was this plate of rotten fish? Well, it was a plate of rotten fish, *Surströmming* to give it the correct name, fermented with just enough salt to stop it decaying totally. Apparently, it had something to do with salt restriction by the Hanseatic League in the middle ages; I confess my concentration wandered. They gave me a tin to take home. On leaving for Sweden I had asked my wife what she wanted me to bring her back as a gift; she suggested Mats Wilander. He was the famous, Greek god-like, Swedish tennis ace of the time, who travelled everywhere with a tin of this stuff, so they said. He was welcome to it.

Over the years I led workshops in Iceland and Finland, but never in Norway, much to my mother's displeasure. In 1994 Hässle paid for a translation of my brand new book, *The Doctor's Communication Handbook*, and soon Sweden was awash with them; they were free after all. But I am getting ahead of chronology and will go back to try to keep a logical sequence. As Søren Kierkegaard said, 'Life can only be understood backwards; but it must be lived forwards'.

In the 1980s and 1990s Russia wanted to join the Western world, and at the instigation of Professor Lesley Southgate from Barts, I was invited to help run a course on doctor–patient communication in St. Petersburg. This was partly because of the recent arrival of *The Doctor's Communication Handbook*, and because of my involvement with the development of the video examination for the RCGP. My co-contributor was Paul Julian, a GP from Hackney, London who had an expertise in running Balint groups, and teaching the lessons learned.

To try to teach communication to any group of doctors is a high-risk pastime, to try to teach a group of Russian postgraduates who speak no English requires an optimism bordering on insanity, or perhaps an arrogance of epic proportions. Paul and I did not feel arrogant or especially optimistic; perhaps we were just stupid. We had been given five days to prepare the programme and then to run it. The Medical Academy for Postgraduate studies of St. Petersburg would provide the participants, and the venue. We were given our flight tickets and were to be provided with a flat each. The pre-course briefing was not too encouraging, with a great many do nots, such as drinking the water, taking too much money, travelling alone, taking expensive cameras etc. We were both apprehensive, and just a little gloomy. I was not looking forward to the experience. How very wrong I was.

We knew the Russians were very into Balint. He was the Hungarian psychoanalyst who had practiced at the Tavistock Clinic in London in the 1950s. He had worked with a group of pioneering English GPs, including my own trainer, John Horder, and got them to study the emotions in the doctor–patient encounter. He coined the phrase '*the drug doctor*' and talked about '*apostolic function*' and '*the collusion of anonymity*', and he wrote a very influential book called *The Doctor, His Patient and the Illness*. Paul was a co-author of the follow up *Doctor, the Patient and the Group: Balint Revisited*. We did not know each other, and I had to play down the fact that Balintian thought was not for me.

It was very cold in St. Petersburg. We were greeted by Professor Yuri Gorbachef and his daughter, Ludmilla, who was to act as organiser of all things that needed it. We drove past the still new Second World War Memorial, followed by the Napoleonic one; there were lots of holes in the road. We stopped at the gold-domed Cathedral. Yuri gestured to tenements nearby, 'Raskolnikov lived there'. There was a little boy fishing through the frozen Neva River on the way into town. We pass a statue of 'Great Peter', and Yuri laughs 'you two, Peter and Paul, disciples I think, but who of?'

Ludmilla tells us her first communication joke. 'I tell my husband I am worried; I went to the doctor today and he says I need blood pressure pills for the rest of my life. Oh, that's no big deal says he, so why be worried? … He only gave me four tablets'.

We arrived at the Medical Institute deep in the back end of St. Petersburg. It is not a pretty place. The restaurant was Lebanese, but utilitarian and gloomy. 'No foreigner would eat Russian food' Yuri said, looking sad and shaking his head. 'We have been divided by five in the last five years, what is to happen?' We feel a tinge of anxiety; we are in a very strange place, with a sketched-out plan for a course that would not cover the proverbial fag packet. Would anyone turn up? What did they expect? The food, we had been warned, was pretty dreadful, but we went out and bought some good wine and told stories. Paul got a telephone directory to contact his Russian aunt. It was a very slim volume and covered all of the city.

Sixteen doctors turned up for the course, about 50:50 male:female ratio, mostly in their 30s. Paul did the introduction and we divided them into trios. Here they could share their experiences and hopes for the course in their own language. There was lots of chatter, laughter and enthusiasm. In truth, Paul and I turned out to work well together, but our Russian was non-existent. How did you run a course in communication skills you might well ask? Katya was the answer. Katya Schlachter was a young Russian doctor, married to a mathematician, who spoke perfect, fluent English. I asked her on day one of the course, when I discovered that she could translate faster than I could think (not too difficult I hear you say), just how she had learned it so well? 'Vorld Service' she replied. She enlarged a little later, by telling me that since childhood, every night she had listened to the BBC World Service broadcasts and learned her English that way. This was a dangerous thing to do in Russia during the Soviet regime, but her father had thought it important, and had believed that a time would come when it would be necessary to know English. I was only the second English-speaking person she had met. The other had been a Jewish professor from the Bronx, and she had not understood him very well! She loved Paul and me because we spoke like her radio.

On the third day of the course, I was staring out of the window, looking at the desolation that was suburban St. Petersburg. It was grey. Huge blocks of identical flats stretched as far as the eye could see. A defunct tram blocked one of the central tracks. The pavements were covered in broken paving slabs and the gap between the flats and the roads was mainly rubble with the odd weed. The thing that really got to me were manholes without lids, oozing steam but with absolutely no protection for any pedestrian, who could so easily disappear down one. I turned to Katya and, with some frustration, asked what it was about her town that made it so unhelpful and unprepossessing to its inhabitants? She smiled and said (I can hear her now), with her deep Russian lilt:

Ah Peter, you do not understand our country yet. After 70 years of revolution we have a saying... 'otherwise it would be convenient'.

The power of that saying 'otherwise it would be convenient' has not diminished. It is such an acceptance of what cannot be changed.

By this time in the course, some things were becoming clearer. Russia was still a mess. Many features of Russian healthcare were strange to us; some bad, some good and some just different. In most countries, doctors are socially and economically privileged, but in Russia a doctor's pay was lower than the average wage, and they earned more 'moonlighting' as taxi drivers. Under Communism, medicine was a poor relation of mechanical engineering. The biomechanical model ruled supreme, and enthusiasm for medical technology, imaging and endoscopy was strong. We learned of a professor, who had an interest in psychosomatic issues, branded a 'non-person', deprived of rights to travel or to meet foreigners. He had wanted to come on our course but was unable to. Despite this, we discovered a rich vein of spirituality in Russian culture that made even worldly-wise apparatchiks open to Balint and the humanist side of medicine, while herbalism and physical therapies seemed fully integrated into Russian healthcare. Methods of medical education had failed to keep pace with developments in other parts of the world. Teaching was mostly by didactic lectures, and postgraduate training focused on defending a research thesis rather than on practical clinical skills. Katya admitted quietly that she was a member of the Anthroposophical Society, strongly influenced by the works of Rudolph Steiner, a heartfelt form of Christian Mysticism focusing on the soul.

Andrei was the oldest doctor on the course by a long way, wearing a very old jacket, and even older shoes. He was a specialist in terminal care, not a common specialty at that time. He had worked with Dr Robert Twycross at The Michael Sobell Hospice in The Churchill Hospital, Oxford, as had I. He said he played bells to his patients and wanted this course to make him tastier to them, his patients.

The course went pretty well until the afternoon of the third day. The participants had role-played a work-a-day consultation and were now discussing the performance of the doctor. The doctor was Timor, a tall, thin emergency doctor with, as it turns out, an even thinner skin. I had not properly stressed the rules of debriefing consultations; good points first, and no criticism without recommendation. The Russians came from a hard school, they were not used to taking prisoners, Timor's nervous and faltering performance was dissected without mercy. Paul and I tried to protect him but we were too late, and the episode left a bitter taste. I have never underplayed the rules since. Vladimir, a submariner from Ukraine, was unsympathetic; he said it was Timor's fault for being useless. It turned out that they were good friends. As I said, it was a tough school.

On the fourth night Andrei invited Katya, Paul, Paul's wife Mary and me to have a meal at his apartment. This was a chance to get the real feel of

Russia. It turned out to be the most bizarre and wonderful evening I have ever experienced, and I retell it as much for me as for you. You will think I am making it up; I am not!

Andrei's flat was in old central St. Petersburg, 15 stations away on the metro, and a walk past an army of indigent poor, selling one onion or half a chicken, all with that same Slavonic look of absolute resignation. This was still a chilling country. Katya kept looking over her shoulder. I asked her why? 'Force of habit' she smiled.

It was very dark, and the apartment, despite the detailed, beautifully drawn map, was not easy to find. A very old babushka helped in the end, and pointed into the gloom towards a sort of fire escape that looked as if it had been built in the time of Peter the Great. We spotted a dilapidated looking lift with a Cyrillic sign on it. Katya translates it into 'Danger of Dying'. We walked; of course, it was the top flat. We knocked on the door, nothing. After a while we knocked again, and the door opened slowly just with the effort of knocking. It was dimly lit, not a bulb over 25 W. There was a hall full of metal dancing figures, thin, Lowry-like, and every square inch of wall was covered with an artefact; a picture, a mask, a sword, a gun, a hat and, wait a minute, was that a shrunken head? Suddenly, our view of this mysterious interior was obscured by a man in a shiny black cape, wearing a top hat and sporting a superb waxed moustache. He swept off his hat and theatrically gestured to come in. There was a gale of laughter, not quite normal laughter, which went on and on. We recognised it; a penny-in-the-slot laughing policeman. Then it was real laughter, Andrei's laughter, the caped crusader. His tiny and beautiful wife Natasha stood, rather apologetically, waiting to greet us. An early clockwork musical box played *The Magic Flute*.

'Oh, my husband. You must forgive him; he is a good man but not right in the head, you understand?'

We laughed and Andrei laughed loudest. There was a mannequin standing in the warm, dark, shadowed, main room, with a black dress and white shawl; 'The Lady of Death' laughed Andrei. Two living ladies, in 200-year-old dresses, are seated in front of very old Chinese screens. A thin man dressed like an aristocrat was hovering over them and a modern-dressed man was taking pictures. Andrei told me he was a psychotherapist. He pointed to a portrait of Napoleon, 'it is very early, before he became Emperor'. There was a hole in it, 'a bullet hole'. I can believe that. Andrei's mother was a sculptress with a religious bent, and Andrei had her beautiful cast of Christ's suffering face. There were three rare, old icons on a passage room wall. I was whisked into a bedroom and given a waistcoat, a topcoat and a tricornered hat. I realised I was in a time machine. Paul emerged dressed as a successful pirate; it suited him.

Andrei could not stop showing us his treasures, and treasures they were. There were 200 hand bells, all with a slightly different note. He played some Bach on them. Then he showed us his old mirror, Venetian and sixteenth century; it certainly looked old and battered. It was magic, said Andrei with a conjurer's wink. On the wall were two portraits of ladies; one black, lady Death, glowering.

'Look in the mirror,' said Andrei, 'she will smile'.

Death will smile? In the Venetian mirror she did, a soft, kindly, sad smile. In a modern mirror; nothing, just Death. The other portrait lady, serene without the Venetian mirror, scowls malevolently in it.

Rummaging under the bed, Andrei pulled out a huge leather-bound book which he opened with obvious reverence. Inside were the most beautiful pen and ink drawings of fairies, ballerinas, elves, dashing mounted soldiers and lips, pages of lips. The style was Aubrey Beardsley, but almost more accomplished, and deeper. It was very hard to explain but the images resonated, I have never been quite sure of Jung, but he would have understood. Jung believed we all have innate, universal, pre-conscious psychic dispositions that form the substrate from which the basic themes of human life emerge. These archetypes are components of the collective unconscious, and serve to organise, direct and inform human thought and behaviour. Jung thought that archetypes hold control of the human life cycle; in this little flat in newly freed Russia it was the first and only time I understood what he was getting at.

'They have all been hidden for 80 years, they have survived like the human spirit, which is why they are important, and they are survivors of a more beautiful time'. said Georgi, Andrei's wife.

Then she smiled patiently and said our supper was ready. Throughout the excellent and simple meal of stew, dumplings and beetroot served with blood red Russian wine, Andrei never stopped talking, relating the terrible things the Russian people had suffered in general, and St. Petersburg in particular. He asked me to guess how many had died in the city during the Second World War. We suggested half a million. His laughter was hollow this time. Three million he told us. Wikipedia might beg to differ, but it was a lot, more than all of us can really imagine.

After the sweet of honeyed baklava, Andrei took Katya by the hand and led her from the table. On the far wall were several metal plates, rectangular and varying in size from two by one foot to about four by two foot.

'These are for my patients, I let them choose which one is for them.'

He tapped a few of them. The intensity and depth of the sound, touching parts hard, even impossible, to touch, was unbelievable. One sounded like the Steppes, another an Anthroposophical soul, a third was made of rocket metal and sounded like 2001: A Space Odyssey. They had ribbons threaded through holes on each side of the plate. Andrei stood Katya by these plates, chose a middling-size one and, with the ribbons, hung it gently over her neck and round her shoulders. He steadied her as she staggered under the weight, then holding her shoulders, he looked deep into her eyes and slowly tilted her forwards until the thick metal plate hung away from her body.

'Stay still little one' he said in Russian, in by far his softest voice to date.

From off the wall he produced a padded hammer and without warning struck the plate with some force, right in the centre. He dropped the hammer and held Katya tight by the shoulders. The sound, such a sound, so unexpected, so soulful, so even, so deep, went on and on. It was like the Russian Steppes, and yet very gradually the note changed and began to fade. I looked at Katya: tears were rolling down her face; not little tears but a flood. Still he held her. The noise got fainter and fainter and more intense. I know that doesn't make sense, but it is how it was. Andrei's fingers were white and buried into her shaking shoulders. Then it was quiet. Katya was quiet too. Andrei relaxed his grip and removed the bell (for that is what it was) in one easy movement.

'I do that with my patients' he said and slumped into an armchair, silent.

Andrei's 14-year old daughter, Anastasia, appears. 'Do you love Tolkien?' she asks. We talk of Frodo and the Ring, of Gandalf and Mordor, and suddenly Mordor seems close. It turns out it was closer than I thought.

We arrived back at our flats, and at around midnight there was a knocking on my door. Paul for a nightcap? No, two large, grinning

Russians pushed in. I took in that they were wearing slippers, so they must be staying here too. They are drunk. They question me in Russian, do I want vodka? No, but that is not the correct answer, and after firm prompting, I say ok. They whoop and one ran to get a bottle, the other opened my drawers to see what I have. A sense of nervousness crept in. The bottle was labelled 'Black Death', the best Swedish I think they say, better than Russian. Was there a threat here? It was like having two half-tamed bears in the room. The bigger one, about six feet four inches, said he was a 'surgeon morgue'. I think he meant pathologist, he talked of bullet holes; the other seemed to be telling me he was a police doctor. I drank a toast with them, in a gritted-teeth, bonhomie sort of way. They insisted on one swallow, they were not small tumblers. Out came the Russian cigarettes, long cardboard tubes with short fags at the end. It was no time to refuse. They liked my name, Peta, Peta, Peta they repeated. Another toast, I tried to refuse, there was anger, the feeling of threat grows and I drink another toast. The wimp card is called for. I said I was tired, and that my heart was tired. I said I have a pacemaker and draw a diagram; the big one was fascinated. I must show him, he felt the pacemaker, pushed on it, laughed, stood up, turned and was sick in the corridor. Obviously feeling better, he came back in. 'Strip' he said. He began taking his shirt off; if I had hoped for a Russian dalliance it was not this sort. This brought me to my feet, emboldened. 'Niet' said I, shooing them out. They hover, I insisted. 'Zaftra?' said one, tomorrow I assumed. Ok said I and manage to shut and bolt the door. Tomorrow never came I am pleased to relate.

The prior warnings about the water supply proved accurate. The St. Petersburg water system was full of giardia, and despite deliberately not drinking the stuff, we were all struck down by day three. The standard treatment was metronidazole, but with that antibiotic's poor interaction with alcohol, it was an unwise choice in a country that ran on vodka. But the show must go on. On advice from Lesley Southgate, we had brought Ciprofloxin 500mg with us and took 1,000mg as a stat dose. It worked a treat. We were even able to lay on a buffet lunch for our diligent course goers, with goodies never seen in Russia at that time, that we had brought from England. I have never had a smoked oyster since.

On the last night we were invited to a medical dinner given partially in our honour. The Russians are parsimonious by learned necessity, and so we shared the stage with a graduate being awarded his PhD, although at least this was an all-medical affair. Paul's wife Mary was to be taken to the Mariianski Theatre to see the ballet. She was extremely happy with this arrangement.

I was sat next to old Professor Yuri Gorbachef, with Katya on my right. We started with a toast; a small glass of vodka drunk straight back in one go. Several more followed! Yuri spoke good English, learned from the World Service too. He asked me if life was good for a doctor in England? I gave him a long-winded version of yes. I asked him the same question. He told me that now it was ok, although not great, and that doctors were not highly prized in Russia. There were a lot of doctors in Russia, but it was better than it was. 'Than it was?' I echoed. He went very quiet, and then I could see that he was crying.

'Just one word' he whispered into the table. 'Just one word. That is all it took. One word in the wrong place and then the Gulag or worse. Yes, there was worse'.

Katya saw what was happening and whispered for me to be careful. I think she really meant gentle. Yuri went on to tell me a common Russian story of a bourgeois family, virtually exterminated by Stalin who hated any sort of intellectualism. It was not a common story to me, and it was so raw to him. The loss of brothers, daughters, parents and friends covered most of the several courses, and many more toasts. The scale of the horror made it almost impossible to grasp, but the look on the old man's face made it real. The Russians do misery very well, but they are also a humorous people, much more so than the Americans, and they had a sense of the wicked. Katya had confided that they actually missed the Communist Party and its stupid rules; now they were gone there was nothing to laugh at.

There was the knife tapping on the glass again, and the host stood up. He was the Dean of Medicine, a big man with a round, squashy face and deep black, twinkling eyes below bushy white eyebrows. He looked like the villainous, twinkling Russian in the early Michael Caine films. He had a voice like melted black chocolate. Katya whispered the translation into my ear. He looked at us directly, thanked us for our services and then said it was a little Russian custom for the guest of honour to tell a joke for the company. He chuckled and fixed me with a gorgon stare. Katya nudged me with her elbow. I was on! This was unexpected, unprepared and deeply unnerving. The brain was rummaging through hundreds of half-remembered jokes in the fraction of a moment it took me to stand and grin inanely at the assembled company. The old ones are the best; the evolution joke came to me. I will tell it to you, but you have to imagine it being instantly translated into Russian.

Two little dinosaurs are happily eating ferns at the side of a lake. Suddenly a crashing noise sounds behind them. The lake ripples ominously to the tread of huge footfalls. They look behind them. Horror of horrors, it is a Tyrannosaur! The first little dinosaur immediately starts running but the second calls after him 'There is no point, you can't outrun a Tyrannosaur'. The little fella shouts back 'No, but I can outrun you!'

Paul came up with a better one, which sadly I cannot remember. But they all laughed, and Katya patted us both on the back. After another toast, the Dean rose again. A bloodstream overloaded with vodka meant Katya's services were much less necessary, as the brain was sort of instinctively processing the language. He looked directly at us again and in his wonderful voice spoke in Russo-English.

'Now I will tell you all a little story'.

To appreciate this to the full, read this out in your best Russian accent.

'This is an important story for our guests, Peter and Paul, who had the good manners to come here with Russian names and the even better manners to help us learn how to improve our medical care in this beautiful city, and to teach us all how to communicate'. He smiled, a deeply ironic smile. 'They came with their foreign language but Katya, our colleague here, translated for us and so we have all learned from our new friends. Well, let me tell you a little story to illustrate the importance of our lovely Katya's skill. In an old house there was a mouse, a hungry mouse. One day a smell wafted into his mouse-hole behind the skirting board. It was a wonderful smell: it was cheese, but such a cheese; the smell so good that the mouse was almost driven crazy. He peered out to see if the coast was clear, but he hears Meeiaaow! Ah, he thought, 'The Cat! If I go out now, she will kill me'. So, he waited. But the smell, it was intoxicating, it filtered deep into his being, he needed that cheese, he must have it. He peered out again: Woof, Woof! 'Ah that is the dog. The dog will chase away the cat and I will have my cheese'. So, he rushed out to have his fill, but he did not get more than a foot. The cat jumped on him and killed him.' He paused and scanned the company. 'The cat, she turned to her kitten, 'Now you understand the need for foreign languages'.

A couple of years later, Katya, Timor and Vladimir came to stay at my home in Culham, Oxfordshire. They were all Tolkien and CS Lewis fans, so the proximity to Oxford was a big draw. But they had a special request, they must go to the next-door village of Sutton Courtenay, and to the graveyard of All Saints Church. Why? The churchyard is the burial place of Eric Arthur Blair (1903–1950), better known by his pen name, George Orwell. As a child, he fished in a local reach of the Thames. He requested to be buried in an English country churchyard of the nearest church to where he died. However, he died in London, and none of the local churches had any space in their graveyards. Thinking that he might have to be cremated against his wishes, his widow asked her friends whether they knew of a church that had space for him. David Astor was a friend of Orwell and was able to arrange his burial in Sutton Courtenay, a 'classic English country village' as Orwell had specifically requested, as the Astor family owned the manor. In 1998 the grave was obscure and minimally tended, but three young Russians were moved to tears. 1984 had been and gone.

REFERENCES

Balint M. 1957. *The Doctor, His Patient and the Illness*. London: Tavistock Publications.

Balint E, Courtenay M, Elder A, Hull S & Julian P. 4 Mar 1993. Doctor, the Patient and the Group. Routledge: Balint Revisited. *Journals of Søren Kierkegaard*. 1843. IV A, 164.

8

The Video Examination: What We Learnt

The video examination ran for a decade, finally defeated by statistics, clunkiness, general irritation and College politics. The RCGP wanted to be the organisation that controlled entry to the profession, which meant using the MRCGP as an entry examination. This also meant a fundamental change in attitude to the exam; it stopped being aspirational and became necessary. You could argue that this had not done much harm to other professional qualifications, such as the Membership of the Royal College of Physicians and Fellowship of the Royal College of Surgeons, but general practice is different. Lord Moran's ghost is still walking in the corridors. The exam had to be toned down, minimal-accepted competence would now be the calibration.

Over the 10 years that the video component was in place, we looked at over 90,000 consultations from around 13,000 doctors. The exam was created around patient-centredness, defined as the ability and willingness to consider the patient as an equal in the communication, to actively seek out their preferences for involvement in decision making, to ask about their ideas, concerns and expectations, and to use these in the explanations, with an aim of reaching a shared understanding and possibly a shared management plan.

WHAT DID WE DISCOVER?

Well, with some notable exceptions, trainees did not convincingly demonstrate what they professed to believe in. In the MRCGP oral viva examination examiners were taught not just to expose the attitudes of the candidate, for or against termination for example, but to seek the justification of that attitude. The argument being that you can't really mark attitudes out of 10, but you can have a stab at rank-ordering the justifications. This is not easy, and one person's justification is another's bigotry. Justifications tend, of course, to be post hoc, cortical intellectualisations of inherently mid-brain feelings. In the oral examination all candidates, without exception, claimed they believed in, and practiced, the patient-centred method, and most could describe several consulting models and the concepts behind them to the satisfaction of the examiners. But in their videos, effective patient-centred communication was rare. It rapidly became clear that candidates' attitudes were not necessarily what they claimed. We can say this with absolute certainty, because we watched so many consultations from so many doctors, and we found that only around 10% of doctors could demonstrate the behaviour of actually involving patients regularly in consultations which they themselves had selected to demonstrate just that. In 1985 Tuckett found the same, as had Byrne and Long a decade before us. We confirmed their findings, in spades as they say.

The most common reason for failing the exam was not demonstrating an ability to involve the patient in simple decision making. Not discovering anything about the patient in a social and psychological sense emerged as the second most common reason for failure. Questioning the patient in an insufficiently observant manner to determine the patient's agenda was the third most common reason. It was quite apparent that doctors really did wish to involve their patients, but found it difficult to do so.

This was a breakdown in the theory; the stated attitudes did not lead to the stated behaviour. The candidates, as that delicious rotter Alan Clarke famously put it, were being economical with the actualite. Modern medical exams encourage candidates to play-act what they think assessors want to see. But does this behaviour carry on back in the surgery? Our video experience would suggest a very definite no. We also learned that good consulting is not a natural gift for most. It needs to be worked at, it must be practiced, and it must be critiqued. Young doctors were already trapped in unhelpful styles, and flexibility over a range was rare. After watching so many consultations we learned that some behaviours you could put your shirt on. When doctors finished the search phase and moved to examination they never went back, never, with 99% accuracy. So, if the search for ideas, concerns and expectations was short, it remained short. Many trainers would not believe me when I told them this, and kept scrolling through their own videos to prove me wrong; it is one of the few times I wished I was a betting man. On reflection this may be the most important teaching point we learned; do not examine too soon, and if you do, please learn to go back for more information.

Contrary to our expectations, there was little or no difference between male and female doctors, indicating that good consulting, by our definition, is a learned behaviour for all. Foreign-born and trained graduates did worse, again with notable exceptions, and UK-born graduates could not be distinguished by ethnicity. What all those thousands of videotapes did demonstrate, most clearly, was the very special relationship that patients have with their doctors. This represents a feature of human society that has existed continuously from the shamans to the present day.

The first, and overriding, aim of this assessment was to put consulting on the academic map, to make it important enough for doctors to study it, and practice it; as I have said, the exam was primarily intended to drive learning. We didn't get it all right, the methodology was cumbersome, and with all the modern technology now available, it would be much easier today. The criteria seemed clumsy to some, and some behaviours were selectively, if accidentally, overused. 'Are you worried that you are the man who put options into general practice?' asked a weary colleague, after watching yet another spurious offering of non-realistic alternatives to a bemused patient.

The odd thing to me is that practicing patient-centred medicine is in fact pretty easy if you want to do it; you just have to listen, be curious and participate in a dialogue not a monologue. But you do have to *want* to do it. After witnessing 40 years of communication courses, models of educational behaviour, tasks, strategies and programmes full of skilful simulated patients, hours of dissecting videotapes, clever skill training workshops as both a trainer and an 'educator', I have seen agonisingly slow changes in actual doctor behaviour. Again why? The simple answer must be that the majority of the profession don't rate patient-centred, evidence-based, shared decision making as worth the time and emotional effort to them, and if they feel like that then all the knowledgeable, clever teaching in the world is going to make no, or at most very little, difference. I had hoped the exam might change things; on reflection I don't think it did.

So, looking back, do I regret the video experiment? Well no, this is a competitive world, and now I spend more time being a patient than a doctor. We were trying to test the real, useful working knowledge and skills of a human being, from the top two per cent of our educational system, who have been through five years university education, and then at least four more postgraduate years of supposed intensive training. I want my doctors to be seen to be competent, and to have had their metal tested by a modern, wide-ranging assessment that still embraces the concept of failure. But I also want them to understand me, and fit their general treatments to the individual that is me. In so doing, I also hope that if their assessment maintains or even improves a standard, so will the profession. Mediocrity is to be fought at all costs.

As the Millennium approached the old gang of four came together again, 20 years after we had started writing *The Consultation*, feeling that we and the world were just about ready for another edition. This rewrite was a more subdued affair, testosterone levels were down, there was much less marking of territory and very little antler locking. A whole year went by without us doing anything. We brought a lot of learned experience to the table. Theo had risen high in the RCGP and was our most experienced conference attender. Peter had organised much of the Oxford Region's trainers' courses for years and, with Theo, had honed a regular consultation training course for two decades. David was now a successful management consultant, running Edgecumbe Consulting with his wife. His interest was drifting away from doctors consulting, and focussing more on leadership and team development. We were all struggling with the fact that patient-centred medicine was proving a lot harder than we had hoped.

In 1998, when we started to write the new edition, two major developments had collided; evidence-based medicine and the concept of patient-centredness. The results of this collision were slow to reveal themselves, but would be seismic, wide ranging and fundamental. A paper by Bensing in 2000 helped clarify some of our thinking.

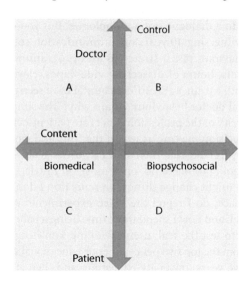

Doctor–Patient model.

The traditional medical style is A. The empathetic paternalistic doctor, who gives their patients plenty of room to tell their own story, but who at the same time is firm about medical decisions would be B. A doctor with a broader patient view, but still essentially disease-based, would fit into C; a common pattern with chronic fatigue patients for example. The doctor with an essentially bio-social view of illness will be D. The interesting thing about this model was where the patient fits. It can be anywhere. Many patients wish only bio-medical explanations. Some want involvement, C, and some don't, A. Patient B is happy with a paternalistic doctor who however takes an interest in them as an individual, whereas patient D is happier setting and controlling the agenda. From the doctor's point of view, the model demonstrated unequivocally that patients are different in what they wish to discuss about their problems, and how personally they wish to discuss it. This meant that the best way to know the patient's agenda was to seek it out by all the communication strategies at the doctor's disposal. This agenda would then help the doctor to seek out the right balance in the decision-making process, and to titrate how much to share and how much to subsume.

The most immediate problem with this advocacy was that in the UK it conflicted with much central advice to primary care physicians. The National Service Frameworks of that time, the vast majority of national screening programmes, and almost all immunisation programmes did not routinely entertain the concept of patient involvement in decision making and, in most cases, actively militated against it. The concept of clinical governance, usually an audit-based, number-crunching exercise, measuring such areas as the uptake of aspirin following myocardial infarction, needed to be modified urgently to take account of not just the evidence-based needs of patients, but their un-evidence-based views and beliefs. We felt that unless the profession was prepared to tackle this increasing divide further, advocacy of improved communication between doctor and patient was likely to be so much hot air.

We stressed that there was an urgent need to change the long-established concept of 'history taking', and to replace this methodology with a structure of communication that values the patient's contributions. Doctors commonly misunderstood what patient-centred communication meant, internally defining it as friendliness, sympathy and professional efficiency, but missing out the essential component of involvement. Doctors needed to be taught that what mattered to the patient, should also be what mattered to the doctor. Traditional teaching had not proved very effective in changing doctors to more participative styles of communications, and new methods must be tried. We began to advocate a teaching-by-questioning style.

In a moment of breath-taking inspiration, we called it *The New Consultation*. It took a surprising long time from the first meeting in 1998 to publication in 2003. I think we remain proud of this work; it has sold over 5,000 copies in the UK, been translated into at least eight languages and remains on many important reading lists. There is no doubt that it was a more learned, but subdued, version of the original. I think we lost a little of the fizz. We backtracked on the 'rules' and still did not venture down the road labelled 'skills', but the video experiment featured prominently. We did wonder if there was a hole in the middle of our philosophy? Were the tasks still relevant, and if they were, were they punchy enough? They were certainly seen as interesting, but old hat, by many. If this was to be the *new* consultation book, should we consider a restatement of tasks in the light of experience? This was the leap of faith we made in the early 1980s and was it time to do it again?

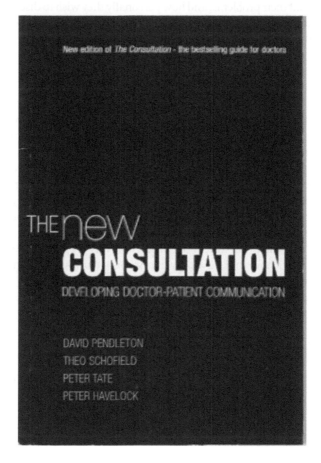

David Pendleton, Theo Schofield, Peter Tate, & Peter Havelock. '*The New Consultation: Developing Doctor–Patient Communication*', 2003.

We looked in detail at task one and knew so much was done badly by so many young doctors:

> *To define the reasons for the patient's attendance, including:*
>   i. *the nature and history of the problems*
>   ii. *their aetiology*
>   iii. *the patients' ideas, concerns and expectations*
>   iv. *the effects of the problems*

It was not one task but several, which might make it an intellectual jumble. I had never liked task two:

> *To consider other problems:*
>   i. *continuing problems*
>   ii. *at risk factors*

This was a nod to other consultation models, but too often actually got in the way of good consulting.

Task three:

> *With the patient, to choose an appropriate action for each problem.*

Task four was my favourite but rare:

> *To achieve a shared understanding of the problem with the patient.*

We had been working hard on 'management options' but with only limited success. And now it seemed more closely intertwined with task five than we had originally thought:

> *To involve the patient in the management and to encourage him/her to accept appropriate responsibility.*

Task six:

> *To use time and resources appropriately:*
>   i. *in the consultation*
>   ii. *in the long term*

was confused by the word appropriately, and rarely done well in observed video tapes. Task seven was perhaps more crucial than we allowed:

> *To establish or maintain a relationship with the patient which helps to achieve the other tasks.*

I had hoped we would take a bold step and rethink the central tenets of *The Consultation* and restate them in a newer and fresher form. Then perhaps people might have listened more. On a personal note, I was not well as we entered the final writing phase and I confess that my memories of writing this book are by no means as vivid as the first time. The first edition was driven by a passionate enthusiasm, the second was more characterised by ennui and an acceptance of the reality.

In the late 1990s Roger was elected as Chief Examiner and, working closely with David Haslam, modernised the examination. The video examination became the lynch pin for a few more years. There were significant groans from part of the training fraternity, but on we went. All was not well in my own world at this time, and times got hard.

My wife Sandra had struggled with alcohol for several years, and by 1996 she was deteriorating. This was awful on so many levels, but for me, selfishly, the worst pain was my own guilt; fêted (occasionally) as an acknowledged expert in doctor–patient communication, but totally inadequate when it came to the crunch. I took over running the household, learned to cook and tried to see that my children were shielded from the worst of it, but I failed absolutely to help the one I loved. Yet another pacemaker wire snapped, it was four or five by now. They couldn't remove them, so they were just cut off and left, and a new one put in. Health beliefs took over; my first idea was that I was too fat. I was concerned about my nagging, angina-like pain, previously, but dubiously, diagnosed as oesophagitis, and I expected that weight loss would make me feel better, and perhaps improve the gout too. Having tried every conventional diet to no avail, this time the rebel scientist in me thought Dr Atkins' low-carbohydrate strategy seemed worth a try. It worked a treat. Within two weeks a youthful feeling returned, the gout went as did the angina, and a stone fell off. Hope raised her dangerous head, and the future beckoned; I could do my job, look after Sandra and keep working with the exam. Ah hubris, always just around the corner. The recently-replaced pacemaker wire was 'tied off' below the skin in the upper right breast. This was no real problem as there was plenty of fat to cushion it (Mae West might have been envious) but as the fat evaporated the wire began poking through the skin. What to do? I had a learned fear of cardiologists from 25 years of interventions and different opinions, and so developed a different idea; it's a breast problem, so get a nice plastic surgeon to snip the wire, easy; done, a quick day case, and no fuss.

I was down to 14 stone now, more energetic than for a decade, and the little grey cells were bubbling away with vigour, now freed from the custard of lethargy that had seemed to be engulfing them. But what are these night sweats and funny feelings in the chest? Over eight weeks of increasing lethargy and ineffective self-treatment, the concern is clear; I know I have an infected wire, but I also know that to treat me properly they will have to take the whole lot out, and this is not an attractive prospect. The likelihood was death whichever option, and I froze. Ridiculously, looking back, while in this state I went with my brother-in-law, professional golfer Phil Taylor, to the Ryder Cup at the Belfry in 2002. By the second day, I was in big trouble and back in my room in the Belfry hotel. I lay in a full, hot bath for 30 minutes to stop the shivering, but still something stopped me from actually doing anything. That evening I managed a sensible, short conversation with Peter Allis, and drove home after the convincing European victory the next day. Eventually, on the Monday, my wonderful registrar Jo Brody took the decision for me; she tells me I will be dead if something is not done soon and checks my CRP, which comes back at 219 (normal <8). Paradoxically, this makes me feel better; it proves I am not skiving. My ideas are that this will be a long job, my concerns are that I won't make it and my expectations are of an extremely unpleasant few weeks. Two out of three of these proved correct.

Let me say that, from the cleaner to the Consultant Cardiologist, everyone was kind beyond the call of duty, but implacable, all of them. They put an IV line in, warned me of six weeks of treatment, said I probably had endocarditis, and that first and foremost the old pacing system had to come out. I tried some patient–doctor communication.

'What was it going to be like to take the old wires out?'
'Think of it as legalised GBH' said my fellow Geordie specialist registrar with a smile.

This honesty quieted me somewhat;

'Er what about the risks?'
'Ah only for old ladies, of course there is tamponade, but the right ventricle is such a low-pressure system that it's no real problem.'

The insouciance of it all. There was no point in whingeing.

'Er the pain?'
'We'll give you what the Russkis gave the Chechens, that'll keep you quiet.'

Well it did, and with added fentanyl, a five-hour struggle felt like 45 minutes, and the vaguely-remembered feelings of tugging, and the heart mildly objecting to being turned inside out, were academic rather than emotional. I later heard that several doctors came from other teaching hospitals to watch; I think they were selling tickets. I did however sort of get the feeling that all was not 100%.

'Well how did it go?' say I brightly, the next day to the
assembled band at foot of my bed; a brief but unmistakeable
dropping of eyelids, shuffling and forced smiles.
'Fine just fine'. There is a strained attempt at humour.
'Shame your scrap value has collapsed'.

My friend, the Geordie, is detailed to come back with a slightly fuller
version of the truth.

'We thought we might lose you, you know' is the opening
gambit.
'I thought only old ladies died?'
'Well yes of tamponade, but it was the IVC (intravascular
coagulation) that really worried us'.
'Eh?'
'Well, like toxic shock, all those wires with toxins on them
being stripped off was too much and it all coagulates and
that's it really'.

My ideas on informed consent were shaken to the core; was I pleased
I didn't know this risk beforehand? I decided that yes, I was, and sank
further into passivity. In the lull that followed the registrar filled the gap.

'Shame the wire snapped'.

I felt like a stunned trout and let the fly dangle in front of me.

'You see there's a fragment we will need to take out'.
'Where?' was the best I could manage.
'Oh, it's just in the pulmonary artery, no real problem. We
had better put you on fragmin (blood thinner) injections
till we fish it out. The interventional radiologists are going
to do it next week'.

So that was alright then. My ideas about fragments of wire in pulmonary
arteries were vague in the extreme, my concerns were also vague but much
nastier, and my expectations of more pain and faffing were about 100%
accurate. 'Fragment' turned out to be a euphemism for two and a half
inches of something that looked like barbed wire, but was in fact a very
frayed 25-year-old wire. I felt inexplicably better for it being out.

'Is that it?' The eyelids drop again.

My concernometer registers 'Oh shit' on a five-point scale.

'Well there is another fragment... stuck in the right ventricle... would need open heart surgery... probably ok to leave it'.

Now, probably is a word for doctors; it is not a good word for patients, but the repartee has dried up. The registrar fills the silence.

'Your creatinine is not too good, too much gentamycin so we will have to keep an eye on the renal failure first anyway'.

Kidney failure and nasty fragments somewhere crucial? A Chagall-like vision of dead, daffy-looking ducks floated by, and the concernometer went off the scale, but no real sound came out other than a sort of John Mills, circa 1945 propaganda film when his leg has just been blown off, comment of:

'Oh, that's a bit of a bugger, ah well...'

I am reminded of Kenneth William's famous rejoinder to the question 'Dammit man where is your stiff upper lip?' 'Above this loose flabby chin'.

All was not well at home. Sandra had taken the opportunity of my being in hospital to stock up on supplies, had recharged her oesophageal varices, and did her best to bleed to death while I was being operated on. The children expected both of us to die that weekend. Neither of us did but it was very close.

There was another election for Chief Examiner, and this time my number came up. This was my proudest professional moment, but the odds of me being well enough to do the job were very long at that point. Weeks went by, I was allowed home to give the IV antibiotics myself; much to the chagrin of the wonderful nurses, who were all firmly of the opinion that most doctors could not be trusted to wipe their noses let alone do complicated injections. I felt better too, except for the angina which had recurred on mild exertion, but my spirits were up, and I was not dead. The agonising gout had gone as the kidney function had improved, and the thought of going back to general practice, my patients and my partners was an attractive one. Repeated echocardiograms showed no concretions, but the tricuspid valve was damaged, and my relative unfitness was ascribed to this. Get fit was the message, and so I did. A good friend volunteered to babysit the very frail Sandra, and I was walking the fells and the Roman Wall at Housesteads for 10 miles on a Saturday in January

2003, when −5°C, and with no angina to speak off. A check treadmill was arranged for next week before going back to work, but that was just crossing the T's. I felt good, no pacemaker for the first time for 25 years, and soon this would all be over and just a story; my concernometer had dropped to far too near zero to be sensible and my expectations were of a busy return. Did I mention hubris?

Even I could see the ST segments were very wonky, but the chest tightness was mild, and I did do nine minutes, however the eyelids were down again. The consultant came and was solicitous and firm:

'Looks like stents ... need angiography PDQ... in fact I have a cancellation, see you tomorrow'.

The ideas about stents are pretty good; it could be worse, and the new antibiotic ones seemed a real step forward. The concerns that it might just be a bit dodgy are not too bad, and the expectations of still getting back to work soon are ok. Another trip through the hospital on my back; I swear I could navigate this hospital just by looking at the ceilings. Much bonhomie followed by silence again, the television shows a picture I don't want to see. Why is there very little white dye getting down that big artery on the left ventricle?

'Peter I am afraid you have a problem...'

Says the kind and slightly sad voice of Yaver Bashir. I think of my father, dead at 57 with occlusion of the same artery. I am 56. Stenting is not possible, there is critical occlusion of the left main coronary artery, and the right system is not too good to boot. All that red wine to no avail. I was fairly fit half an hour ago, now I am an invalid facing another major heart operation with all the uncertainties entailed. He won't even let me go home because the narrowing is so critical; bleating about walking the Wall is just wasting breath.

'Peter, which cardiac surgeon would you like?'

Being a GP I know who I don't like; coded responses pass between us. He smiles and says he would recommend the youngest, who is a good communicator; a further smile, almost a wink. This suits me fine, but being a patient I want him to be the best operator in the UK, and don't really care if he is ruder than Sir Lancelot Sprat. Ah, how values change.

As it turned out, Chandi Ratnatunga did a great job, and me a great favour. He grafted four cardiac arteries, opened up the heart while he was at it, and removed a large piece of what looked like shrapnel. I don't think my valves would have lasted long if it had stayed there. There had been talk of putting a pacemaker back in, but he didn't, and I have now had 16 years without it. I often wonder if I ever really needed it, but without that experience would I have gone down the path I did?

There is no further suspense in this story, as you know that I made it. Sandra didn't, dying miserably in my own cottage hospital not long after. I was hit with a total body fatigue, which was probably as much mental as physical, and my partners were understandably pushing to know when they could expect me back. The truth was that I did not have the energy to do a good job with my patients so, on genuine medical advice, but with an enormous sense of guilt and sadness, I resigned. I think my partners were relieved, and I have never been back. Soon after all of this I met Judy, was fed up with being miserable, and remarried. Fortunately, my children encouraged me, and life since then has been much better than I deserve.

Mothers know the truth about you and use it when necessary, mine used to tell me that I liked the sound of my own voice. I was an only child, loved facts and liked arguing, so I talked to myself a lot. Not having an imaginary friend, I had a doppelganger that lived in my head, with ideas and views that were unwise to give free rein to. Is this a split personality? My time lying in a hospital bed gave me the space at last to read Freud, and about him; the man who really started all this doctor–patient communication stuff. I knew what he had helped to create, this self-indulgent, self-obsessed and overly introspective world, but still don't know what Freud believed, not least because he kept changing his mind. He was conscious of his Jewishness from an early age. On entering the medical school in Vienna, he researched the sexuality of eels. At the time these creatures were linked to Jews and Gypsies because all three had strange migration patterns. Truly! He spent weeks trying to become famous by being the first to discover their testicles, and he failed. This slimy episode put him off the gorier aspects of medicine, and he turned his not inconsiderable intelligence to more cerebral matters.

He became very interested in cocaine, and poisoned one of his best friends with it, but his real goal was to help patients bring repressed thoughts and feelings to the surface. In 1896 he said that the symptoms of hysteria, until then a madness thought to arise in women's womb, actually derived from sexual abuse in childhood, and claimed that he had uncovered such incidents for every single one of his current patients (one-third of whom were men). He lied. If you read his papers and letters from this period, it is clear that these patients did not report early childhood sexual abuse as he later claimed. According to Freud, people often experience thoughts and feelings that are so painful that they cannot bear them. We can all empathise with that. Such thoughts and feelings, and associated memories, could not, he argued, be banished from the mind, but could be banished from consciousness. Thus, they came to constitute the unconscious. This was his repression theory. In explaining the Oedipus theory Freud said:

> I found in myself a constant love for my mother, and jealousy of my father. I now consider this to be a universal event in childhood.

I had always felt he was the creator of a complex, psychological web which has been acknowledged by too many as real, without even a glimmer of testable evidence, which perhaps is one of the great follies of Western civilisation. In creating his particular pseudoscience, Freud developed an autocratic, anti-empirical intellectual style. Let us face it; he was a charlatan. In 1896 he published three papers on the ideology of hysteria, claiming that he had cured a number of patients. First it was 13, and then it was 18. And he had cured them all by presenting them with the fact, or rather by obliging them to remember, that they had been sexually abused as children. In 1897 he lost faith in this theory, but he had told his colleagues that this was the way to cure hysteria. Therefore, he had a scientific obligation to tell people about his change of mind. But he didn't. He didn't even hint at it until 1905, and even then, he wasn't clear. Meanwhile, where were the 13 patients? Where were the 18 patients? You read the Freud-Fleiss letters and you find that Freud's patients were leaving at the time. By 1897 he didn't have any patients worth mentioning, and he hadn't cured any of those he had had; which he knew perfectly well.

You will have gathered Freud has never been a hero of mine, and I still think that he contributed more than his fair share to the development of the society we have become. I can write this now because what I think no longer matters in a consulting room. Undeniably, he was a clever, brave, irascible and eternally curious man, who spent the latter years of his life trying to prove that the iconoclastic, long-skulled, monotheist Pharaoh, Akhenaton, was in fact the biblical Moses. He may even have been right about that, but he certainly was not right about the interpretation of dreams, or the mumbo jumbo that became the religion of psychoanalysis. When Judy and I visited his consulting rooms in Vienna they were packed, and the visitors were obviously awestruck, behaving as if in a religious building. I have heard it said that Americans passed from barbarism to decadence without the intervening civilisation. There may be some truth in the statement, and dear old Sigmund had a lot to answer for there. It was America who took his ideas to her bosom and then exported them back to the Old World, who never accepted them quite so uncritically. After all I have said, there is a bit of me that still likes him though.

And what of the exam? This was less onerous a job, and with encouragement I did my term as Chief Examiner, retiring in 2006, and as is my wont, not going back. I was popular with the Panel and I still wear the Omega watch they clubbed together for, but the world of the exam was changing, and my sympathies were out of step with the political movers and shakers. I still wanted a genuine hurdle, wanted the calibration to be above minimal competence, but the times were against this. The video days were numbered, and simulation was to be the order of the day. Regular sampling showed that yes, the exam cohorts were improving year on year, but the young doctors really did find patient-centred medicine very hard to do, and although we could demonstrate change in behaviour, it was not as dramatic as some of us, especially me, had hoped. I did regret the passing of the old and the over hasty adoption of the new, but then, as Mandy Rice Davies so famously said, when the cabinet minister denied, on oath, having sex with her; 'Well he would wouldn't he!'

REFERENCES

Bensing J. 2000. Bridging the gap. The separate worlds of evidence-based medicine and patient-centered medicine. *Patient Educ Couns* 39(1), 17–25.

Freud S. 1897. Letter to Wilhelm Fliess.

Pendleton D, Schofield T, Tate P & Havelock P. 2003. *The New Consultation: Developing Doctor–Patient Communication*. Oxford University Press.

Tuckett D. *Meetings between Experts: An Approach to Sharing Ideas in Medical Consultations*. Law Book Co of Australasia, 19 December 1985.

9

Career Reflections

What is wisdom? I keep hoping that, as I get even older, it will strike me. So far, no luck, but here is a bit of what I have learned, medically speaking.

Most of what I was laboriously and expensively taught at medical school in the 1960s was wrong or, at best, not right enough to be really useful. My medical house job was at Sunderland General Hospital, full of little Durham miners at the far end of the long ward, wheezing their last shallow breaths, while smoking a home-rolled tab that glowed brightly from the oxygen they were on. We could do nothing useful for these wonderful, coal-soaked men. In the rest of the ward the nurses were spoon feeding heart attack patients lying flat on their backs for 10 days, while fiddling with the next-door patient's milk drip to 'cure' his duodenal ulcer. He was probably a manager at a local shipyard who was constantly under pressure. He would smoke 20 Senior Service a day, and the nurse adjusting his drip would think him a typical type A character whose ulcer was basically his own fault. Anyone suggesting that his ulcer was actually an infectious disease would have been laughed out of court. 99.9% of all known experts agreed, until an extremely brave (and, or, stupid) Australian doctor called Barry Marshall swallowed a jam jar full of a very nasty bug called *Helicobacter pylori*, in an effort to prove that stomach ulcers were not caused by stress and bad diet, but by an infection. The profession had laughed at him, but he was right, and in 2005 was awarded a Nobel Prize.

There was a nearly-forgotten Dorset farmer who did something similar, and was hounded out of his village of Yetminster for his pains. During a smallpox epidemic, he injected his family with cowpox, believing it would protect them from the more virulent virus. He was right and they survived. 20 years later, country GP Dr Edward Jenner repeated this technique, took all the credit and invented vaccination, which led directly to the absolute elimination of the smallpox virus 200 years later. Ponder that for just a minute. Academic learned consensus has a life of its own, it feeds on itself and is harder to attack than Genghis Khan, but in many cases is in fact as vulnerable as the Alamo.

Among my main jobs as a house officer were adjusting digoxin doses to control heart failure, now considered to do more harm than good, working out insulin doses from urine tests, a truly mystical art at best, and dishing out gargantuan amounts of antibiotics, but not to ulcer patients. One relative blessing was that the 'Crash' trolley was very rudimentary, and death was mostly a lot more peaceful. My father, paradoxically, had a better armoury than I was to have. He could give really effective antipyretic doses of aspirin to children, a much, much more effective drug than the now ubiquitous, and glutinous, paracetamol. There were real antispasmodics for colic, gripe water that could get you banned from driving, sedatives that really did sedate and cough mixtures, loaded with opiates, that you could stand your spoon up in, and gave genuine relief, unlike today's expensive placebos. And while on that subject, he used placebos quite openly with the time-honoured red, green and black bottles, and to good effect. He did not do much screening, and was not inclined to treat epidemiological, asymptomatic risk factors. South Shields may have had an increased death rate, but can you show me an individual who felt aggrieved? Health beliefs were different then too, based on expectation and experience. You can't wish for what you don't have, you can't expect what isn't possible, and concerns were more fatalistic. It was only two decades since the end of the Second World War; South Shields and Sunderland had been bombed to smithereens, and this altered health perspectives. I suspect we are living through another major shift and it will take some time for the dust to settle.

And what are we left with? Modern communication between a doctor and an anxious parent for example is now seriously weakened. Take the anxious young mother to start with. Her ideas: my child is unwell, he needs urgently checking by a doctor. He is distressed, and in pain, and these need relieving as quickly as possible. I think he has an ear infection because he is pulling his ears a lot. Her concerns: my child might be seriously ill, could it be meningitis, could it be COVID-19? She is concerned too that you might not take her worries seriously and will make a mistake about the severity of the illness. Her expectations are clouded by her worries, but include the idea of a curative prescription, the possibility of a hospital admission and the difficulties of getting to, seeing and understanding doctors.

Now take the doctor's understanding. I am assuming for this example to work that we are past the pandemic. Your ideas: this child is the fifth hot, cross, under one year old you have seen today. What does mum expect of you? This is probably a self-limiting illness caused by a germ whose name you hope you don't know, but as most childhood infections just get better, the likelihood is that this one will too. Your concerns: this mum is distressed and angry, is it just because of the illness? Is the child really ill? How much reassurance can you give? Your expectations: Mum will want antibiotics but needs educating not to expect them for all childhood illnesses. If you get it wrong, you know she may call out-of-hours later tonight.

The consultation starts badly because of mum's difficulty getting to see you; you go on the defensive and try to soothe things down by examining the cross child thoroughly. This reveals nothing except pink drums, probably caused by screaming, and a temperature of 39°C. The stark truth is that, other than reassurance, you have nothing to offer. Mum may interpret this as bloody-mindedness, or professional negligence; a wilful withholding of cure and protection that her distressed child so manifestly needs. You may crack, providing the amoxicillin, and perpetuating the saga. Research suggests that ascertaining and coping with mum's concerns is the most effective way of dealing with such consultations, but that for many the only way to do that is by antibiotic prescribing. So, what do modern doctors do?

You have antibiotics that don't work, but parents want, and have lost, the old weapons; placebos and magic. You still have caritas, but sometimes our patients don't believe that. The science has replaced the art, and in so doing has lessened your ability to treat and manage minor illness. I can see why both doctors and patients turn ever more to alternative therapies, unproven and silly though many of them are. They at least offer the magic of healing.

Health beliefs have changed dramatically over my lifetime, as medicine and society changes, not always for the better. Life is more complicated, there is more choice, often too much to really make sense of. Informed choice is an ideal, but it is more often than not a will-o'-the wisp, seen fleetingly but never actually grasped; this makes most attempts at informed consent very difficult, and in many cases genuinely impossible. As a counter to this not-often-admitted fact, consent itself has shifted from a noun to a verb, as in the consultant's instruction to the junior, 'Go and consent Mrs X for her operation tomorrow'. This is not a sharing; it has become a procedure.

In an attempt to extract a limited form of wisdom from my coal face experience, these next few anecdotes are going to be excruciatingly honest. They relate to feelings I have had about past experiences with patients over an extended timescale. In any human relationship much is left unsaid, assumed or not admitted at all; the doctor–patient relationship is no different. The fact that better outcomes usually result from patients trusting doctors is an accepted truism, though for all previous centuries it was more likely to harm than heal you. Even today, the effectiveness of 'alternative' pseudoscience and quackery, such as homeopathy, chiropractic, osteopathy, ayurvedic etc. looked at dispassionately from a sceptical, battle-hardened old medic perspective, is almost solely down to a placebo effect, supercharged by trust in the practitioner. What happens when you turn this conundrum around? How much should doctors trust their patients? We know uptake of medical advice is poor, the rule of thirds holds true, but what about trust at the relationship level, the stories people tell us, how true are they?

Continuity is not an unmixed blessing, for doctor or patient. It often leaves huge lacunae of ignorance about people you have seen regularly over an extended period. After 30 years attitudes have fixed, ears have closed and patterns have become preordained; being able to recite the probable patients and their complaints for one's evening surgery before even looking is an amusing game to entertain bored receptionists, but perhaps symptomatic of a developing malaise. I confess to never knowing patients as well as they thought I did, and sometimes after 30 years of regular contact my knowledge of the real life of that human being in front of me was pathetic.

After I had been in practice a decade I shared, as it were, an early middle-aged female patient. She saw my senior partner mostly, but when he was away or just unavailable, I was the reserve. We both thought we knew her pretty well; she was a blousy barmaid at a local spit and sawdust pub, her mousey husband was a cabby and she had two early-teen children who did not help the police with their inquiries too often. Her council house was neat and clean with a well-tended little front garden. We both thought her a pleasant, unremarkable and uncomplicated citizen. The medical problems she brought to us were humdrum and quite usual. Then the police called and asked to see us both at the end of a morning surgery. She had been found murdered in a bus shelter down by the Thames and could we tell them anything medically that might help the perpetrator be brought to justice? We were aghast and perplexed simultaneously; why would we know anything that could be useful? The Detective Inspector looked at us quizzically, with a faint air of exasperation; we did know she was the town's most popular prostitute? We didn't, but everyone else obviously did. The Inspector shook his head and looked at us with a pityingly disappointed expression:

'Call yourself family doctors, and you don't even know what one of your regulars does for a living'.

We had no answer.

Then there was, let us call them, the Barnes family. I became involved with this family very early on, and still am, sort of. In the 1970s, the town council created its own Gulag, a group of run-down, post-war prefabs hidden four miles away from the town in Tubney Woods. This was for the recidivist families that were considered trouble; non-rent payers, socially disruptive and unable to fit in with middle-class morality, as Alfred Doolittle would have said. Needless to say, it became a GP's nightmare; if the phone went requesting a visit at 3am on a Sunday morning it was odds on that the call was from Tubney Woods, from one of the few unvandalized phone boxes. There were no mobile phones then or, for this enclave, any private phones either.

The Barnes family called a lot. Barry, the dad, was a wicked scamp with a twinkle in his eye who I found it hard to dislike, but who spoke like Brad Pitt in the film *Snatch*. A volume of words that implied you understood all the nuances of his meanings, but in reality I understood little, and the manner of speech made it very difficult to get any clarification. The implication was always that he was a much-misunderstood good guy whom society had judged unfairly. His wife was quiet, stoical, subservient and loyal, to what definitely turned out to be a fault. They had a brood of young children, mainly girls. Over many years, I got to know them all as well as anyone. They moved closer to town, and Barry got a form of religion, and treated himself to a dog collar. Social services called several case conferences on the family in the late 1980s and through the 1990s. There was the strong hint of emotional abuse, neglect and faint, very unsettling rumours of other sexual forms of abuse; even some sort of secret society involved in procuring children. I confronted Barry several times as best I could, and always received indignantly verbose denials. When I got his wife, who I trusted more, on her own she was invariably, fiercely, supportive of her husband. One of my partners who also saw the family a lot was much more damming, convinced that Barry was a dissembling, evil man, and that he wouldn't trust him as far as he could throw him. In the end a very determined female detective got on the case and hounded Barry until at last, only a few years ago, she built up enough evidence to convince the Crown Court, and Barry now languishes at Her Majesty's pleasure. Just before the trial, when I was retired and living in deepest Dorset, a note fell through my door. It was from Barry, mysteriously asking me to meet him at the local pub at a specific time. Very Le Carré, and despite my wife's advice I went, and there in the alcove was Barry, his wife and one of his daughters. He had gone to some lengths to seek me out, and his trust in me remained absolute. By this time, I had known him nearly 40 years. One of his daughters had at last broken ranks and accused him of childhood sexual abuse, his wife and other daughter were still both adamant that this was rubbish, inspired by family feuds and jealousies. What could I, his old family doctor, do to convince the court he was innocent he asked me? Nothing was the short version of a difficult and long conversation. And I don't know the truth; the evidence given to the court had much conviction, my old partner gleefully sent me a copy of the Oxford Mail, and yet here was I, ex-Chief Examiner, with a definite weakness in the trusting department, still unsure.

When we chose and trained examiners for the old oral examination, we found they very roughly divided into three types. Types who were limited in their ability to explore topics, but nevertheless seemed to make consistent, and reproducible, judgements in line with other information on the candidate. Types whose questioning was forensic, but whose judgements were out of line, and types that seemed to be good at both skills. There were hawks and doves in all three categories, iron fists in velvet gloves and gruff, grumpy Gradgrinds who passed everyone. The ones we rejected were the ones whose judgements were consistently out of line; we had discovered that you could not effectively train for this skill, it is innate. I wonder about my own skills, waiting as we all do for that officious little man to knock on the door and tell me that I have been found out.

There is another family that has a very similar story. I looked after the mum, Francis, from the time I started in practice; she needed regular monitoring because of long-standing medication for chronic and severe mental health problems. I saw her through her two pregnancies, and always had a slightly tricky relationship with her innately aggressive, and fundamentally layabout, husband. The years went by, there were case conferences here too, all centred on possible neglect and physical, but not sexual, abuse. One daughter in childhood manifested a wide range of quite severe, but ultimately psychosomatic, illness. At one stage in the late 1980s I wrote 'CARE' in capitals in her case notes, suspecting that we were missing a deeper and more unpleasant truth, and her condition worsened to the extent that in this daughter's early teens she was taken into care and improved quickly. All this was before Jimmy Saville. As a society we were not as alert to sexual abuse as we are now, but professionally we were slowly waking up. Again, I probed, cajoled and questioned Francis over several years to see if she suspected anything untoward in her husband's relationship with the daughter. There was never the faintest crack in her vehement denials. The police became convinced but could not get the evidence. I could not provide corroboration, but I was more convinced than in Barry's case. The husband took my lack of corroboration as support, which was difficult. Not long before I became ill and retired, I met the daughter in the town. She stopped me, said that I had never believed her, but that her father had consistently abused her over a period of several years, and that she was certain that her mother knew. As you can tell, this encounter haunts me still. To my recollection, and borne out by the case notes, she had never suggested to me that she had been abused despite direct questioning to that effect, but later she had to others. The same dogged detective got on to me a decade later, and again the jury were given convincing evidence and he too is in prison. I gave evidence to the court, and when I arrived, the father in the dock smiled and waved, perceiving me a friend; he still trusted me, but I did not trust him.

And then there was Margaret, who I mentioned in Chapter 3, and after sending back my young trainee to diagnose her MI we became friends, in a solid doctor–patient relationship, but not social, sort of way. This friendship lasted nearly 25 years, when she at last remarried and moved away, only to return after a couple of years. I was very pleased to see her again; we were old friends and I was saddened to hear about the death of her husband. I was well aware of the poor circulation in her right leg, as I was involved in her first arterial graft in 1977, which itself was a complication of cardiac catheterisation, following another MI diagnosed by myself. The leg gave her intermittent trouble for many years; she even had a pet name for her leg, and she continued to smoke. She eventually had an emergency popliteal bypass, complicated by an MRSA infection. I noted, not long before she left, that her peripheral vascular disease was severe, and I, the great sharer of understanding, was convinced she knew how precarious the circulation in her leg was. When she returned, I noted 'pain in leg, ischaemic, slightly worse because had stopped nifedipine. Death of spouse while away'.

She came to see me in the surgery a few weeks later. I have a copy of my actual note, the consultation lasted 18 minutes. I have entered: 'Foot pain really getting severe again, right foot and calf cold, chat re recognising and trying to avoid gangrene'. It is my recollection that during this encounter we shared the possible options, and that Margaret was aware of my opinion that there was no further surgical operation that was likely to restore her circulation, and that with care and drugs, amputation might be avoided in the short term, and that it was justified to wait to see if the collateral circulation could sustain the foot. She had feared amputation since 1977, and I was trying to help her keep her leg for as long as possible. I thought she was involved with, and understood, this strategy, but was wrong. I prescribed oramorph for the increasing ischaemic pain, with clear instructions for her to call if this was not controlling her pain, or if the clinical signs in her leg were changing. After a few days she acknowledged that the situation was now untenable and requested immediate referral to the vascular clinic; there was a clear understanding between us that this would mean amputation. She was seen next day in surgical outpatients, admitted and the dreaded but inevitable amputation ensued. I saw

Margaret several times after her amputation until my own illness in October 2002 forced my retirement. On none of these occasions, when she often called me Peter, did she complain about my handling of her case. Then, as you have probably guessed, five years after retirement I received a formal solicitor's letter complaining of inadequate care. This was the last thing I would have ever wished, as we had in fact been close friends for over quarter of a century. I felt her graft had virtually occluded even before her return, and that amputation, which she herself so feared, was the likely end point, but that conservative treatment was justified until the clinical signs or the pain became intolerable. I was also convinced, obviously incorrectly, that she both understood and shared this management strategy. My then-new wife Judy could not understand how such an action could come about and was distressed at how upset and gloomy I became. It was a sort of assault on my own integrity and core professional beliefs. Many of my friends have had very similar experiences and have spoken of the disproportionate disturbance and sadness such complaints produce. In this case, a single letter from me with the factual details was enough to hear no more, but the sadness and self-doubt remains.

When thinking about long-term relationships, it was Michael Balint who first highlighted the innate problems with, then much less common, repeat prescribing. His point was that, after a while, the doctor–patient relationship sort of became a truce. The various arguments have been heard on both sides, and a sort of status quo reached, exemplified by the repeat prescription. When this stage of dynamic equilibrium had been achieved, there were reasons for both parties not to rock the boat too much. Particularly with psychoactive or painkilling drugs; the patient had achieved their aim and there was little incentive for the doctor to interfere, as to do so would produce a deluge of new consultations until the equilibrium was restored. Although many modern checks are in place to try and monitor repeat prescribing, these observations remain as valid as 50 years ago.

My last registrar asked me, not long before she left, how I could remain so calm and apparently understanding with Barbara, who was forever in the surgery, and had the most complex and hair-raising repeat medication list of opiates, antidepressants and anxiolytics. I set off on the explanation as to why Barbara had reached the state that she was now in.

At time of our first meeting in 1974, Barbara was 26, attractive, vivacious and married to an ambitious young accountant with prospects. I supervised her normal pregnancy and even delivered her of Tom, a small, noisy baby, via low-cavity forceps for delay in the second stage; this was in the long-since defunct maternity unit in the local cottage hospital. Delivering babies, in some cases more than the act of procreating them, seems to produce a sort of bond between people. It was to be so with Barbara and me, but sadly Tom soon showed signs of heart problems. He failed to thrive, remained a slate-blue colour, and the heart sounds were non-specifically abnormal. He was transferred to the local teaching hospital, and then for further investigation into a specialist unit in London. It slowly transpired that he had a severe congenital abnormality of the pulmonary artery, along with some other defects, and that his prospects for living past infancy were slim. Barbara and her husband were understandably hit very hard by this news, and Barbara became depressed; this deepened over some weeks until she needed hospital admission without Tom, who was looked after by her husband's parents. She made a slow, shaky recovery. After her discharge, I visited her at home several times, as was the norm then. She confided that she did not want to love Tom too deeply, as the pain of his dying would then be too much to bear, and that she felt guilty about having these feelings.

This situation never really resolved, and the years went by. Tom did not die in infancy, and by the age of five was a strong-willed, very intelligent little boy, fiercely angry at the constraints on him placed his own body and, as he saw it, his overprotective mother. Bill, the husband kept getting promoted. Barbara was in a state of constant hyperawareness of every breath Tom was taking, and constantly trailed the little lad around every specialist in the land, receiving many different opinions but no help. She was convinced a heart transplant would be a solution, very reluctantly accepting that even this would not cure the anomaly buried deep in the lungs, and then that only a combined transplant would do; which at this time was not an option. Tom however carried on living a disabled, fraught, but very contributive existence. Wherever he spent time he made an impression, leaving his mark on carers, teachers, friends, doctors and, indelibly, on his family. Seven more years passed, Tom had frequent collapses that threatened, but did not lead, to death; Barbara carried on searching, smoked constantly and developed a series of intractable symptoms too long to list. More and more doctors became involved, and their care became increasingly fragmented.

Then, finally, Tom's valiant heart began to fail, and both parents wanted him at home. His final illness lasted a week and I visited two to three times a day. With advice we gave him sedation to ease his obvious suffering, but Barbara nursed him constantly, cleaning him, giving him drinks, always trying to comfort him. It was breakfast time one morning while I was visiting, when Tom sat up, stared into his mother's eyes only a few inches away, screamed 'I hate you; I hate you', and fell back dead. There are silences and then there are silences; this was the second sort. Bill pulled Tom's lifeless body to his chest and sobbed convulsively; Barbara didn't move and stared out of the window. I couldn't trust myself to speak and was effectively useless, just able to touch Barbara on the shoulder in a pathetic gesture of sharing her pain. A minute, or an hour, went by, and then the room filled with a slow moan, starting soft and melancholic, building over aeons to a screaming, high-pitched wail of such intensity and pain that I can hear it now. It had not been easy initially to localise the sound to an individual, but by now Barbara's head was thrown back, and she was shaking both Bill and the departed Tom. The sound wouldn't stop, perhaps it still hasn't.

Weeks later, Barbara confessed to me that Tom was haunting her. Standing by her bed, rotting and accusing her with hate-filled eyes. My psychiatrist friend had a name for it, but the image haunted me too. Gallons of platitudes were poured on Tom's unkind death, bucket loads of 'you did your best, you have nothing to reproach yourself for' type of remarks, streams of 'you know he didn't mean it', but Barbara nearly drowned in her river of grief.

Barbara's severe distress was exhibited by extreme illness behaviour. Freud would have termed it '*hysterical conversion*'; a more modern, but ugly, word would describe it as '*somatisation*'. It seemed that her overwhelmed coping mechanisms tried, as a last resort, to fight fire with fire; or in her case pain with pain. She started the round of specialists again, low back pain and pain in the kidney regions being the main symptoms. Several esoteric diagnoses appeared, some seemingly dependent on the amount of money changing hands. Her private medical subscription was soon enormous. Various strategies were adopted, and drugs were added to her cocktail on a seemingly random, haphazard basis. None of them worked but they became needed, and the need escalated; paracetamol became dihydrocodeine, became morphine and finally heroin. Anxiolytics went from diazepam 2mg, to 5mg, to 10mg, to lorazepam, and the same with antidepressants. 10 years after Tom's death, Barbara was still in pain and taking what she could for it, and Bill was still doing his best to cope, but thinking of early retirement. Over 10 doctors and at least 10 other professionals were involved with Barbara but who was in charge? Balint's famous collusion of anonymity was being starkly illustrated. I tried, honestly, I did, and a few times we managed meetings of Barbara, Bill, myself, the pain specialist, the psychiatrist and the cognitive therapist. We adopted strategies, created rules that were always broken, but always for understandable reasons. The partners got more and more upset when I was away at having to provide repeat prescriptions for regimes that they were profoundly uncomfortable with. Barbara, conscious of this pressure, over-ordered lest she ran out, but in so doing her consumption went up, fuelling the addiction, increasing the pressure and magnifying the disapproval.

It was at about this stage that my registrar asked me how I could remain so outwardly calm about this pressure for drugs, therapy, care and attention that seemed all but insatiable. The truth is, the calm was the outward manifestation of an inner guilt. It is all very well to say that if you know everything, then you will forgive everything (this phrase sounds much better in French by the way, *tout comprendre c'est tout pardoner*) but forgiving isn't solving. I was guilty that my understanding and my forgiveness, however hard-won, had not actually been enough to prevent the life-destroying medicalisation of a human being I genuinely cared for. I wasn't the only health-care professional who had failed, but I was the lynch pin, the coordinator, and to assuage my guilt I acquiesced to most of Barbara's requests. My partners understandably thought this was taking a profoundly unhelpful, easy option and objectively they were right, but at the emotional level I wanted to make amends for Tom's death and my own inability to help relieve her suffering. Over the years this frustration even came out as anger, the glacial calm sometimes being replaced by petulant frustration surrounding repeat prescription requests. GPs who know and forgive may still not improve your health, and continuity may not always be for the best, but it usually is.

Doctors, like people everywhere, prefer an easy life to a hard one, so there is a temptation to keep seeing the patients you like, and restrict the ones you don't. This can be difficult in partnerships when one partner consistently fills their surgery with chronic repeat attenders meaning that all the urgent acute cases have to be seen by another; this in my experience has been a very common reason for partnership grievance, even leading to breakdown. Doctors and patients becoming friends can be a highly charged relationship; it is usually fine but there are many, many examples of it not being so.

The medical circumstances of friendship formation can be dramatic, as was the case with Harold. He had moved from France into a huge, Addams Family-type house in the mid-1970s. Soon after moving in, he became acutely and frighteningly psychotic, and I was called. On arrival in my open top MGB, built of course in Abingdon, a gesticulating, sixtyish man in an ill-fitting tweed suit ran out of house, shouted something unintelligible and proceeded to run rings round my car, still shouting. An elegant, tall, slim lady, who turned out to be his wife came to me, shooing him away and allowed me to get out. There was a tear in her eye, and the fact that her husband was acutely crazy did not need a medical opinion. What to do was the question? By now he was picking up large rockery stones and dropping them in the fountain. He needed to be restrained, and the only legal way to do that was to section him under the then terms of the Mental Health Act. This was prior to the major improvements of the

1983 Act. He needed a senior psychiatrist in a hurry; this was usually a big ask but not this time, and within a couple of hours Ben Pomryn, Oxford's first community psychiatrist, arrived. I have mentioned him earlier, but this is the time that we first met, and I became good friends with both of the major players in this tale, until both died, far too soon.

By the time Ben arrived, Harold was getting even madder; he told me later that he was trapped in a living nightmare, genuinely dreaming, half-knowing it was dream but the demons were so real, and the irrationality was totally logical in a dreamscape world. He needed sedating, restraining and hospitalising. In those days I used paraldehyde by intramuscular injection. I had used it in similar circumstances while a ship's doctor. It is horrible stuff, must be used with a glass syringe as it dissolves plastic, and is a very painful injection with a high risk of causing abscess. But it is safe in the sense that it does not cause respiratory depression, can if necessary, as it was here, be injected straight through a tough pair of trousers, and is the most effective sedating agent I have ever used. Of course, no one ever uses it now. Ben agreed with the strategy and sat in his car while I got on with it; that is the hierarchy as it was. Although a big man, I was a bit nervous at that time that in any struggle my new pacemaker would be displaced, but sometimes you just had to get on with it. After a period of shadow boxing, his wife Odette persuaded him to embrace her, and I did the deed from the rear. He was not happy with me, it must have been very painful, but within a very short time he was on his knees, then lying down and soon snoring. Ben produced a straightjacket, the ambulance arrived and they took him off to Littlemore Mental Hospital.

It was some weeks later that he was released. When I heard he was home I went to visit him; we did that sort of thing then. In conversation, I learned he had been the Managing Director of a famous company's French division, until his increasingly erratic behaviour had earned him early retirement, but with lump sum and full pension. Hence being able to afford this ugly, big pile of a house. What was clear to me was that he was still not well; he looked gaunt, the diagnosis was schizophrenia, and he was on large doses of chlorpromazine. Odette joined the conversation and emphasised that the hospital had been kind, but deaf to her suggestions that he was not just mentally ill but physically ill. They had done a few tests, come up with nothing much, said his blood pressure was too high, but that his GP would sort that out, and said this sort of psychotic illness could produce weight loss and illness. There was something not right; I was never the best diagnostician in the class but I was not the worst, and that sixth sense that we were missing something was strong. In his bedroom I stripped him off and examined him thoroughly; his legs were wasted, his blood pressure high at 200/110 and he admitted to increasing weakness which had stopped him playing tennis. The injection site was still painful, for which I apologised, he giving me a rueful smile. The most conspicuous finding was his mottled suntan; curious. A distant bell ringing. Was this new I asked? He obviously hadn't given it much thought, but on reflection thought yes, perhaps. Nowadays, with the help of Dr Google, I would have typed in wasting, psychosis, high blood pressure, muscle weakness and vitiligo; in those days the old internal thinking machinery had to do it. I wondered; it could be couldn't it? Was this President Kennedy's illness, Addison's disease, an autoimmune adrenal insufficiency? Well it was, and rapid admission to a local private wing, attention by one of the clever Oxford physicians and an ACTH (adrenocorticotropic hormone)-stimulation test proved the diagnosis conclusively. Treatment with titrated corticosteroids rapidly restored him to good health, and the Largactil was thrown in the bin.

He was grateful, and invited my wife and I for supper. He produced some good wine and admitted the real reason he had bought this house. It had a huge cellar, a rarity in modern English houses, and he had a huge wine collection going back many years. His one stipulation at dinner was that we should talk about the wine, stressing that that was what it deserved; each bottle was unique, had a story and should not be just gulped down without a passing thought, except that it tasted quite nice. Sandra did not really buy into this, liking the drinking but not the discussing. Harold sussed this immediately and when the second invitation came, it was just for me. This became a regular, monthly event for around three years; Odette would prepare a cassoulet, confit or similar and then fade away while Harold brought out a wine and told me its story. Then an apricot tart, crème caramel or cheese with no biscuits would appear, and out would come a dessert wine, with another story. It was always a French wine, usually at least a decade old. Harold believed all wines, whether cheap or expensive, white, red or sparkling, improved with careful ageing. His favourite word was the French 'terroir' which he believed was essential to the enjoyment of wine. It is a vaguely understood word, at least by me, and not a scientific concept, but is at the heart of wine's dual appeal as a drink: one that not only enhances the mood of its users but that also derives its enduring sensual characteristics from the physical surroundings in which it comes into being. I was soon a passable expert in a field of dunces; Harold liked claret, my palate liked the mid-Rhône, and he introduced me to Gigondas, superior in many ways to the nearby, and more famous, Châteauneuf-du-Pape, which he thought not worth drinking under 15 years old. I paid for my taxi there and he paid for it home. We did try to extend our friendship away from the wine bottle, a few nights playing backgammon together at the pub nearby, but wine was the enduring link.

Even now, a good bottle of French wine makes me think of him. Then he died, quite suddenly, I can't remember what of. Cause of death is a curiosity but, without a good autopsy, often a pure guess. Older doctors are very suspicious of statistics collected from death certificates; they have filled in too many themselves. We all remember with a shudder Harold Shipman's creative genius.

A patient's severe illness and dying leave lasting impressions on doctors, sometimes more hopeful and happier than you might think. Andrew has left me an unforgettable memory. I knew him at around the same time as Harold in the late 1970s. He lived geographically at the other end of our practice area, in a village where we had a branch surgery in the senior partner's house, so were considered the village doctors. Villages are different from towns, in the sense of involvement, the all-pervasive, intense web of gossip and the judgements of any action, often harsh. Andrew was then about my own age and part of a clan that was interconnected to most of the genuine workers in the village. He was renowned for being a bit of a Jack-the-lad; so far, he had managed to dodge matrimony but had a succession of girlfriends too long to list.

His problem, when I first met him, was the early stages of Hodgkin's lymphoma. Even then, in the late 1970s, his chances of a full recovery with the latest therapy were considered excellent by the relatively new Oxford oncology team. The then treatment was a combination of four drugs, mechlorethamine, vincristine, procarbazine and prednisolone, and probably some radiotherapy, though I can't remember the specifics. He was a thin, quite tall man, with penetrating, dark eyes, and an irresistible, cheeky smile. He was pretty upbeat about the diagnosis; his latest love would be forever, and he hoped he wouldn't lose much time off work. It should all have ended well. His first treatment session was unpleasant, the nausea lasted for days, some of the sparkle left his eyes and he dreaded the next course, which was worse. Before the third time he came to see me, a different man, trembling, sweating and with an overwhelming dread of what was to come. I rang the oncologists, who had a little of the wimp attitude I myself had experienced, suggested some therapy already tried, and urged me to make sure he came as his life depended on it. I dosed poor Andrew with diazepam and persuaded him to the best of my ability of the necessity to persist. To his credit, he did attend, but it was the worst experience of all, and he was quite ill for days. A couple of weeks later the hospital rang to say he had not attended his next session; I rang his home and his mother answered. She was evasive, distressed and found herself between the rock of respecting Andrew's instructions and the hard place of knowing his actions would in all likelihood be fatal. He had decided, finally and categorically, not to have any more therapy and he did not want any more medical involvement.

In villages you learn where people go. Andrew liked the decrepit, but quaint inn in the quiet centre of the village; with prior information I sought him out and found him in a little alcove with his girlfriend (the source of the information). My attempts at persuading him to restart therapy were rejected forcibly, his now fiancée was in tears, and I did not know what to do. It was Andrew who decided; if it was his life, then it was his death, he argued. He now accepted that as an inevitable consequence of his decision, which he stressed again was immutable. He seemed to look at me afresh; it was my job to help him medically wasn't it? Well, as I couldn't help him to live, would I help him die? At first, I misunderstood and mumbled something about medical oaths and respecting life, feeling mealy-mouthed as I said it. Initially he was cross; there was a thin veneer of bravado, but the frightened, confused young man underneath was plain to see. After a while with a sparkle at last coming back into his eyes he shook his head.

'I am not asking you to kill me Doc, I just want you to make my death easier. Can I live a bit before I die?'

Over a couple of warm beers (the barrel was near the fire) we devised a gentle, Faustian plot. When, as far as he and I could tell, the reaper was getting close, I would attempt a timescale, with all the uncertainties that entailed, and increase his prednisolone dose to give him a short boost. He would then set his plan into motion, book the village hall and have a going away party. He wanted to be at his own wake. And marriage? His fiancée had left by this stage. Shaking his head, he demurred, and with a reflective and knowing smile, said it was best he died a bachelor.

It was not that long, a few weeks perhaps, and we both knew then that the downward spiral was now unstoppable. He was emaciated, skin the colour of old scrolls, but curiously animated, almost happy and with a definite sense of purpose. The hall was booked for the Saturday night, invitations sent to all his many friends, for the big bash that was Andrew's farewell. He made it, 120mg of prednisolone daily for a few days helped, and the whole village came. I was invited, and actually drove past, but just could not quite bring myself to join in; there was a thin, almost invisible, professional line that I couldn't cross. By all accounts, he had a truly great time, dropped me a sardonic little thank you note, stopped his prednisolone abruptly as instructed and died within 48 hours. Andrew's was the best death I experienced.

Flora Thompson's *Lark Rise to Candleford* was a must-read in the 1970s. Her honest, but rose-coloured, history of a poor, local hamlet was enlightening and enjoyable. Her apt observation that the medical pedlar's yearly visit was a sell out for period pain medicines, bowel remedies and rheumatic problems, and that after the medicines ran out so did the complaints, remains a favourite. She did however skirt round one of the darker pastimes in isolated Oxfordshire villages. Incest is a very difficult subject, seldom talked about, usually treated with a nervous sniggering guiltiness and quickly glossed over. Forty years ago, it was still a regrettably common social phenomenon. My own prolonged exposure to such a family began soon after joining the partnership. I found a note to visit Mrs Strange because of post-natal problems, having been delivered of a little girl a few days earlier. I asked my partner how to reach the house, and he suggested that I would find the visit interesting, but refused to expand. The house was not easy to find; very isolated on the fringe of a village I had never heard of, but surely did not suffer from light pollution. I was met at the door by a tall, unkempt man with long straggly hair, a sort of Uriah Heep demeanour, and whose main features were huge, riveting, penetrating eyes. The smell was far worse than Mabel's as he led me through a cluttered hall. It was a tip, by far the worst I had seen so far. The kitchen was epically dirty, a month of unwashed dishes, pans and crusted implements. There were fresh-ish plates on one end of the long draining board, and there were dirty ones on the floor; at a glance the system seemed to be that the new dishes at the left pushed along those already there until they fell off the far end. He saw me staring.

'Wife's been out of commission what with the baby an' that, it's all built up a bit'.

We went into a ground floor sitting room cum bedroom, dark, musty, fetid and foul. There was a muslin curtain screening a small camp bed contraption, and lying on it was a frightened teenage girl holding what appeared to be a very large baby. I was not expecting this, and realised my rookie mistake of not reading the notes beforehand. I had, of course, assumed that it would be the baby's mother behind the screen. In the cloying gloom there was another female figure on the opposite side of the 'bed'. I addressed her, the wife/mother, and asked her the nature of her problem. She looked puzzled, and murmured something in deepest Oxfordshire that I didn't quite catch. I turned to the dad for help. He said the mum was having tummy pains and still getting some bloody discharge, so I suggested, looking straight at her that she swapped with her daughter and let me examine her. No one moved. Total naivety; gradually my brain processed the reality, the daughter was the mother. The medical issue was straightforward, though dad never strayed out of sight even during intimate examination, but I still had not fully cottoned on. Trying to make rapport-building conversation with this terrified young woman, I gently asked about the baby's father. She gave me a pitying look, pity for me not her, at the depth of my ignorance. I don't think I really understood until later.

Mr Strange followed me out and I gave him a prescription for his daughter. He said he would follow me in his three-wheeler, but taking my arm, took me to a little shed outside. Inside were myriads of moths and butterflies. He took me to another outhouse with boxes of beautifully displayed pinned butterflies, smiled and told me with some obvious pride that he was the top breeder in Oxfordshire. The full implications and sheer ghastliness of what I had just witnessed was still percolating through my brain, and yet here was this awful man showing me his butterflies.

'Well that will haunt you for a while' said my partner on my
    return.
'Did you see the other daughter?'

On my shaking my head, he continued.

'She is two years older and has a three-year old. There is a son about 14, but you never see him. Quite something really, that bastard has five children by three different mothers, all living in the same cesspit. By the time that little thing you have just seen is in her teens she'll be pregnant by him too!'

I would like to tell you he was wrong. Edith, the experienced health visitor, was sad but useless. What about the police? Well, they had been involved, but there was a wall of silence from the family, no formal complaints and no DNA genetic evidence was available in those days. Over the years there was the occasional case conference, but mainly concentrating on the poor sanitation. The children were fed, went to school and were immunised; their parentage was just gossip.

A decade or more later, I got to know the son, John. He had his father's eyes but not his proclivities, and he had moved away. Not that far, but to a different village. I was a better doctor by this stage, but still carrying the guilt of my inaction. During a surgery visit for something routine, there was an opportunity to touch on this shared, but unspoken, hidden truth. Immediately there were tears in his eyes, and it all poured out. A young lifetime of trying to protect his much-loved sisters from the predations of their father, and shame at the tacit approval of his mother, who saw the father's sexual interest in the daughters as a relief from unwanted attention to herself. His own guilt at leaving was a huge burden, though he was by surreptitious means in regular contact with the sisters, and yes, he was worried that the grandchildren were now coming to an age to be at risk. Then an even darker story emerged, there was a similar family in the same hamlet, looked after by another practice, and the two fathers were drinking buddies, sharing an interest in butterflies, and sadly in daughters too. There had been 'sleepovers'. The concerned horror writ large on my face was shrugged away. The other man was now in gaol, convicted of incest, but Mr Strange remained unjudged. He died not long after of lung cancer, leaving a complicated legacy of love and hate.

Some of general practice was darker than anything Leonard Cohen could come up with, and I have indeed been a Fortunate Man (John Berger), but part of the price is living with the memories of one's own inadequacies, professionally and personally. Most doctors have a warped, black sense of humour, and perhaps you can see why? My own later anxieties centred on an inability to gauge people accurately; everyone who comes to a surgery expects to be listened to, cared for, diagnosed, treated appropriately and preferably not judged. To function, doctors over the years become less and less discriminating in their reactions to their patient's beliefs; it is easier in the surgery to agree. Political and personal bigotry is nodded through; my fear was, and remains, that it was easy to lose sight of what was good, not very good and through and through bad. To be effective it was not my job to disagree, but I fear I did not react well enough to genuine evil, even when I knew I was amongst it.

A final, very sad story to end this chapter. It is the early 1980s, Debra had been my patient from a teenager, and was now a young, married mother of one little toddler. She had a face Botticelli would kill for, and had all the trappings of a successful middle-class life, but she was not happy. In fact, she was distraught. She had fallen in love with a man at work and her life had become a living nightmare. A story as old as the hills, but not one that fits easily into a medical model. The medical school lecture on love was missing, the textbooks are silent, and coping with emotion, as an only child, public-boarding school boy, was not an obvious strength of mine. We had just discovered ideas, concerns and expectations, and I thought this might help her. I sought her ideas; she thought this might be a passing fancy, that perhaps she could have a clandestine affair, that her husband did not excite her but was intrinsically a good man. She was concerned that any affair would be discovered, in any potential break up that her child's future happiness would be harmed and that she dreaded the social stigma that would attach to her. She expected that she did not have the nerve to make the break, even if the lover wanted it and ultimately, she thought she would just have to knuckle down and get over it. I gave her some antidepressants, and arranged a safety-netting follow up. A week later she was different, it was as if she wasn't quite in the room; the psychological term *dissociated* would be an accurate description. She had a bombshell to present, her lover had proposed marriage, given a sort of ultimatum and she realised she had to make a choice, but every option had major flaws. Her love hormones pushed her one way, while her frontal lobe fought against them. How could she make a choice? 'Why ask me?' an all-at-sea, inner voice shouted silently. She was asking me because she trusted me, yet I thought it an unfair question. I suggested she made a list along the lines we had already discussed, with the for leaving her husband in one column, and against in the other, and to come and see me in a few days without taking an irrevocable decision. The next morning, she was found dead in a local beauty spot, sitting in her car still with the engine running. There was a hose from the exhaust through the rear window.

After retirement I left my practice and have never been back. It turns out I was not one of those GPs that could live with the ghosts.

10

Where Does All This Leave Us?

With my recently renovated retrospectoscope, I wonder why patients are so difficult? There are several reasons that come to mind; they are human beings, they are all different, they don't really trust doctors as much as they pretend to, they don't really hear too well and they usually don't do what the professionals want them to. After 5,000 years it is the doctor's role that has changed. No longer the mystical keepers of occult information, the job is now to interpret health information more than give it. The task is to help our patients understand, and to allow them to make valid choices about their own healthcare.

The practice of medicine is a manifestation of the society in which it is studied. My knowledge and practice were based on mainly western, Judo-Christian values, with only the most limited glimpse of other ways of thought. Everybody has beliefs about health, but what they do with those beliefs is culture-specific.

Late in my career, I had an unhappy time in Dubai. A Muslim desert country with golf courses, pretending to be something it isn't. We were advising the appropriate medical bodies on how to introduce the MRCGP examination into the country to help achieve some standardisation of family medicine. Some of the major issues were the values that underpinned the simulated surgery (which has now metamorphosed into the Clinical Skills Assessment (CSA), the assessment that replaced the video examination) and the video examination. These are, of course, an acceptance that valuing the patient's viewpoint, seeking out their beliefs, sharing understanding and involving people in their own diagnosis and management is a good thing. Many doctors in the Emirates could sign up to that, in my experience mainly the female ones, but many others were profoundly uncomfortable with these concepts. Having observed the then current examination in paediatrics, which seemed to be solely the province of female doctors, and when asked to suggest improvements, I remarked that it would be better if the children could see their doctor's faces. I was never asked back. The RCGP's long-term involvement with the extremely rich, but repressive, Kingdom of Brunei has only recently (2019) fallen foul of similar divides in belief systems. The figures show that, in 2010/2011, four years after I left, the failure rate for international graduates taking the CSA component of the MRCGP was 63%, compared with nine per cent of UK graduates. A clear clash of cultures.

It is not just society that influences the practice of medicine, but the understanding of the science of the time. This is a given, but no one seems to give too much thought to the very thin ice on which our overall understanding of the world is based. Even the most educated of us find our understanding of physics effectively stopped with Newton and Einstein, over 100 years ago. Quantum theory, derided by a puzzled Einstein as 'spooky action at a distance', followed by Heisenberg's fundamental uncertainty about everything and Schrödinger's metaphysical cat, clean bowled all but the tiniest fraction of scientists, and even now no one understands the nature of matter, reality or consciousness. This has taught me over the years to treat all medical certainty with a large pinch of sodium chloride. Obviously, we must work with what we have got, but humility is a necessary attribute for a career in medicine. The science is not settled but fluid; at any one time we know some actions are more likely to produce better results and we have to go with that. But it is not Holy Writ, and it changes constantly. My medical textbooks from university are mainly now just silly, my father's were naturally worse.

Doctors and patients alike really dislike uncertainty, it is the biggest problem young doctors face on entering general practice, and people like me make it worse by advising a sharing approach; sharing what? Well uncertainty of course. This is where our complimentary colleagues have the edge; they eliminate uncertainty, there is always an explanation for why the therapy did or didn't work. Always be positive, never show doubt. My dear, I am glad you are improving, let us increase the dose of the Baked Beans. Don't worry that you have not improved, let us use the very special sun-dried African Beans handpicked in the Kalahari. I am sure we can help you if we just cut the amount by a tiny amount, i.e. right dose, or too much, or too little, or the wrong sort. Proper doctors should use the Baked Bean Model sparingly, not least because most of the time they won't have the conviction needed to make it work.

Musing on the nature of human intelligence may offer some insights into the nature of communication. We have found no fossil trilobites with big brains, and they were around for aeons of geological time. Then the wonderfully big dinosaurs ate, fought and farted around (literally) for a huge time span without ever finding the need to develop smart phones. So why, in the last few seconds of geological time, have we evolved intelligence? Looked at dispassionately, intelligence has not been an unmitigated success. We can destroy ourselves on a scale undreamed of in the animal kingdom, and with our capacity to meddle on a large scale, we can now destabilise our planet even quicker than the vagaries of the cosmic forces that surround us. Human scientific progress is happening on a scale so fast that it makes no sense when compared to the relatively slow pace of evolution, even in human history. After all, since 'intelligence', progress is certainly not relentless. Those wonderful and esoteric Egyptians came from nowhere to instant technological wizardry; the Great Pyramid is still literally unbelievable, the second pyramid impressive but not as good, and in no time, they couldn't build them at all. They could still mould King Tut's awe-inspiring funerary mask 1,000 years later, but they carried on going backwards slowly for another 1,000 years until Cleopatra finished it off for good. I remember going to the Tutankhamun exhibition at the British Museum in 1972 several times, as I lived just around the corner in Southampton Row, and after studying many of the artefacts became convinced that we were going backwards, not forwards. The dynastic Egyptians thought that themselves and referred to 'Zep Tepi', the first time, as a time of greater knowledge and harmony.

There is increasingly convincing evidence that an asteroid strike or solar flare reset the development of the human species only about 12,500 years ago, a time referred to as the Younger Dryas. Memories of an abruptly-terminated Atlantean age still haunt our collective consciousness and could explain the profusion of megaliths scattered over the whole planet. The real problem is that we are not clever enough, our much-vaunted intelligence is pretty superficial, and to understand things at all we have to reduce complexities to simple building blocks, thus distorting the true nature of the phenomenon. The number of blocks gets nowhere near the mystery of the Great Pyramid; an equation cannot describe the beauty or the mind-numbing infiniteness of a Mandelbrot fractal. A Manchester rating scale cannot do justice to the subtleties of doctor–patient interactions, and a deep understanding of the Krebs's cycle doesn't help most doctors to cure anyone. On top of this, we become ridiculously possessive and overbearing with the bits of knowledge we have gleaned. Take health professionals. Cholesterol is bad for you, as is too much fat, smoking is anathema and obesity is a dangerous state. All such statements have some truth in them, but take no account of values, human instinct or experience, and the truth is much more complex, multivariate and capable of being viewed from many perspectives. Health messages become reduced to little more than slogans, and the complex, instinctive nature of human decision-making is unacknowledged.

We have evolved to make decisions about situations and our fellows almost instantly; we are often attracted to another across a crowded room, sometimes we dislike on site. We know from personal experience that our original impressions are mostly, but not always, confirmed. Human conversation is based on previous experience, unconscious observations, pheromones, feelings and hunches, but most of our teaching isn't. We are a funny bunch, opinionated, aggressive and irrational, but forever vaunting our intelligence. We all learn how to communicate from a very early age, and most of us are not taught in the conventional sense. When our teachers do attack us with subjunctives, gerunds, past participles, split infinitives and tell us we can't boldly go, some of us are instinctively irritated, some of us make it a lifetime study and most just put such grammatical pontifications to the back of our mind, to be remembered in exams and interviews but not important in our daily existence. Doctors, by the selection methods adopted by our society, are considered intelligent. This is frightening, as all of us have met very stupid doctors, professors and CEOs. In my time as a GP, I was regularly out-thought and out-maneuvered by patients without even an O-level in carpentry. In fact, some of the cunningest individuals I have crossed swords with have, at some stage in their lives, been labelled 'educationally subnormal'. Hans Jürgen Eysenck, remembered for his work on intelligence and personality, postulated cancer types, and heart types. He was the psychologist most frequently cited in the peer-reviewed scientific journal literature, but Eysenck's work has undergone re-evaluation since his death; he was frighteningly close to eugenic arguments and in 2019, 26 of his papers were 'considered unsafe' by an enquiry on behalf of Kings College London, basically for adjusting data to suit the hypothesis; that cigarettes did not cause cancer for example (he was funded by the US tobacco industry). This is a big blow to the pseudoscience of personality types being able to predict outcomes, such as the poorly-validated, psychoanalytically-derived Myers–Briggs test. Within the medical consultation, locus of control is as far as I would seek. Internal control and fatalism have not been significantly linked to intelligence.

So how can doctors consult well?

Rule one: Get the medicine right.
Rule two: Don't forget the first rule.
Then......learn to cope with uncertainty.

This is not easy. Attitudes are crucial; it is the wanting to improve that is the necessary shift. Then the next fundamental step. Learn to listen properly, be curious, encourage a dialogue, share ideas, options and decisions. Doctors must learn to take the rough with the smooth, to keep calm and stay professional; this needs lots of practice, trying of new strategies, more practice, getting feedback. Then even more practice. It's like learning an instrument to a concert orchestra level; it does not come naturally.

Belief systems, or patients' attributions of illness, are crucial to understanding their health-seeking behaviour. Simplifying these beliefs into the trilogy of ideas, concerns and expectations, still a concept I remain proud of, allows doctors to glimpse an understanding of their patients' motivations. This understanding can be used to improve satisfaction and adherence with medical advice. The teaching of these skills to doctors has not been easy, and has become too complex; drastic simplification in teaching methodologies is required. Let me suggest when debriefing a student or junior doctor these questions should be asked:

Tell me what you learned about this patient as a person?
What interested you?
What really mattered to them?
Tell me some of their ideas and beliefs?
What did they expect today?
What was your working diagnosis?
Did you use what they thought when you started explaining?
Did you give them the opportunity to be involved in decisions?
How?
Did you explore their understanding of the treatment?
How?
How do you know that they really understood about the
*   diagnosis?*
Did you agree on (1) the diagnosis, (2) the management,
*   (3) the follow up?*
Have you recorded the salient information?
How long did it take you?

Different initiatives, lockdowns and quality strategies have played hell with doctor–patient communication. The MMR, and now the wider child immunisation debate, has released a Pandora's Box of medieval superstitions mixed with pseudoscience, and not all of this on the patient's side; COVID-19 has only made it worse. The carefully built wall of trust has had a large hole blown in it, and the ensuing gale is threatening the very structure of the patient–healthcare relationship. Some of the conflict, for that is what it is, relates to the 'greater good' argument. The population's health versus the individual's; the arguments, the perspectives and the implications are quite different when viewed from the public health strategy room at the Department of Health, or the worried parents overdosed on a diet of partially-digested internet information sludge, and the high-calorie Daily Mail-omania.

The big question is, in this increasingly hysterical yet constrained climate, is it still possible to do and to train for reasonable patient-centred best practice? The real conflict is between patient involvement, choice and achieving targets. Maybe every 85-year-old should take five tablets a day to keep their blood pressure and cholesterol down so that they can totter on until 90; the trouble is many of them would welcome a quick MI, but perhaps not a stroke. As a patient, this would not be too onerous a strategy, and fulfils Kingsley Amis's dictum, that no pleasure in life is worth forgoing for an extra two years in a geriatric home in Weston Super Mare. But if we don't immunise our children, then back come the diseases. Patients really don't like too much choice; all the worry over potential but rare side effects clouds the issues; and the reality of life, that choices, options and facts are often brutal, is missed. If you don't like the potential side effects of the treatment, then would you rather have the disease? Now you choose or worse, the government will choose for you?

The trouble is that illness in frightening; severe illness can be terrifying. To the extent that the realisation of the implications shuts down our ability to respond appropriately to modern healthcare. Patients were more frightened than I often realised, and mostly thought that their condition was more serious than I did. Many patients were probably mildly afraid of me, and often tended to be passive, and not say very much. This did not mean, however, that they did not want to know what was going on; often I must have missed that.

Most modern patients, but not all, want to be involved at least to some extent in their own treatment, and to understand what is going to happen to them. They have not come about liver or thyroid disease but have come because of the effects of, and their worries and beliefs about, their perceived change in health.

At the coal face I tried to remember, whenever possible, to put myself in their shoes, knowing the goal of merely satisfying patients was a poor one (let's leave that to the alternative brigade), but satisfying our patients is important because we know that satisfied patients are more likely to follow medical advice. Surprisingly, there is little evidence that extending consultation times makes much difference, but communication and style *do*. It seems to be the case that warm, friendly doctors are more likely to satisfy patients than cold, business-like ones. In the jargon, 'positive affect' works well. It also appears that doctors talking too much reduces satisfaction, whereas the sense of being listened to and understood increases it. So, smiling, being friendly and actively listening will mean that patients will often accept some of the less pleasant health messages without becoming fed up.

Patients are just people like me. They deserve respect, they need to be informed and they need to consent. However, people are all different. They respond to a change in health in different ways, and they need individual, personalised plans. All of us can easily have inappropriate and unhelpful illness behaviour reinforced by poorly thought-out and unexplained investigation and treatment. Patients will follow surprisingly little medical advice, unless a genuine effort is made. But they trust doctors, they really do, but not always in the way doctors think.

All of us want to make sense of any perceived change in our health. The GP may be the first person who hears that story, and it may not make much sense if squeezed into the 'medical model'. People come for guidance, advice and treatment. Reasonable health promotion is ok, but stepping over the line into overzealous lifestyle advice is a common pitfall. Most people are less informed than I gave them credit for, and I was bad at remembering that many procedures and screening programmes required much more sharing of understanding than I usually achieved.

Out of the mass of research work on communication with patients, the following stark research truths haunt me. The amount of explanation that a patient receives is directly related to their intelligence as perceived by you, the doctor. The lower the patient's social class, the less explanation is offered. Yet all patients from the highest to the lowest and the brightest to the more intellectually challenged want as much information as they can assimilate, and in a form that they can understand.

The current enthusiasm for shared decision-making is a logical development of the earlier concept of informed consent, itself a relatively new and transatlantic concept, having been first mentioned in a Californian Supreme Court in 1957. There is no doubt that in our present society the idea of informed consent remains very important, very necessary and relates fundamentally to the ability of the medical profession to communicate well with patients. However, looking at the history of medicine, these ideas are remarkably new. The fact that informed consent and shared decision-making are now such major issues is good for patients, as they are offered more information than ever before. Surgeries overflow with leaflets on every conceivable subject, hospital outpatient departments have printed sheets on most known diseases and procedures, but the main driver of this change has been the internet. There is more medical information readily available on the internet than we could ever know, and patients are increasingly more curious, and more inclined to do their own research before presenting to the doctor. This means that patients enter the consultation with very specific ideas, concerns and expectations; GPs are now often seen as the enabler, or conduit, to the investigations or treatments that the patient already knows (or thinks they know) that they need. If patients do as recent NHS guidance tells them, they may already have spoken to 111, a pharmacist and consulted online NHS websites and apps before even arriving at the GP's door. Doctors all need to be prepared for how different the consultation can be with a very informed, opinionated patient, who will sometimes know an awful lot more about their condition than the doctor does. This is a challenge and makes it much easier to lose track of the patient behind the opinions. The real crux of the whole informed consent debate is that to obtain true informed consent requires the achievement of a shared understanding, and a shared management plan. This further implies that the patient's beliefs should be known, and their understanding checked effectively. The ethical imperative behind achieving a shared understanding is respect for the individual. There is an assumption that consent can never be truly informed, so that it is for doctors to determine what is in the patient's best interest. However, health is mainly the subjective experience of an individual and is made up of highly personal beliefs, feelings and experiences. It follows that, when helped by doctors to achieve a comprehension of the risks and benefits of various treatments, it is patients, and only patients, who can really determine which therapy will help them to achieve their most important health goals.

Most consent is a long way from being informed. The internet contains information ranging from medical fact and accepted practice, to myth, supposition and downright falsehood. Most leaflets, while factual, are not very good, some are very poor and some make no sense at all. The moral here is that useful information presented in an inaccessible way is useless information. Information will mean different things to different patients depending on their health understanding, and what is readily understandable to one will be incomprehensible to another. A signature of consent may just mean that the patient trusts the doctors, not that they genuinely understand what is to be done to them and what risks there may be. Doctors are still very influential people, and we must use this influence with care.

True consent is increasingly regarded as a right, and if this right is seen to be denied or infringed, litigation ensues more and more frequently. It may be that informed consent is already an outmoded concept, and that instead patients should be encouraged to actively request a particular form of treatment after having been adequately informed of the options. This request shifts the onus on to the patient; the consumers of healthcare take responsibility for their choice. This behaviour was unheard of as late as 1994 when I wrote the first edition of *The Doctor's Communication Handbook*.

In many areas of healthcare, consent is taken for granted because the obvious benefit of the intervention obviates any dialogue. Much of the screening and prevention industry works on this premise. In fact, it is often nothing more than a cycle of deceit and half-truths; consent is fudged because true understanding is not easy even for doctors, let alone patients.

There is a major ethical divide between a patient visiting for an opinion and help with their agenda, and imposing a screening agenda on that patient. To initiate such a procedure there should be conclusive evidence that the test is likely to alter the outlook for that individual favourably, and that it is most unlikely to do any physical or psychological harm. These issues must be faced honestly, and patients encouraged to ask searching questions. The possibility that screening may have harmful or negative effects is not often considered. For example, in order to obtain true informed consent for cervical screening health professionals should consider doing the following:

a. Inform women of the limitations and disadvantages of the test.
b. Inform women that the absolute benefit, to them as individuals, of their participation in the screening programme is extremely small.
c. Inform women that currently screening accounts for part of the GP's income; there may be a conflict of interest.
d. Check to ensure that women understand the issues.

A study looking into the screening for bowel cancer using faecal occult blood made a startling discovery, which adds further insight into the implications of truly informed consent. In the published study, they randomised those with a lower level of education into groups, and in two groups they used decision support aids which clearly explained the procedure. The study revealed that those with more information reported that they knew more, made more informed choices, and found the decision easier to make than those who did not receive further information. The surprising finding was that fewer of the educated group decided to take the test. The deeply depressing editorial accompanying this paper suggested that 'adherence' might be better achieved by 'a policy of informed uptake rather than informed decision making'.

At last there is hope, Fiona Godlee:

'The Rapid Recommendations team has now taken up this issue, asking whether screening makes an important difference to health outcomes, and which screening test is best. Their methods will be familiar to regular readers but are worth reiterating, because they offer a fresh approach to

providing trustworthy and timely guidance. Triggered by new evidence that is potentially practice changing (in this case, updates from three major randomised trials), they convene a panel of experts that includes patients as full members (in this case, three people who have experienced screening for colorectal cancer). All panel members are required to be free of relevant financial conflicts of interest. They systematically review the evidence and develop guidance, taking a range of transparently described approaches to deal with gaps in the evidence and to incorporate patients' values and preferences.

They find that screening does not reduce all-cause mortality whichever test is used, but it does reduce cancer specific mortality. Acknowledging the uncertainties arising from the lack of strong evidence, they recommend that screening be offered only to people with a risk of colorectal cancer of 3% or more, as assessed by tools such as the QCancer calculator (qcancer.org), and that the choice of test be left to the individual's personal preference.

This personalised and risk-based approach may seem obvious(!!!). But it represents a radical shift, says Philippe Autier in his linked editorial. Screening programmes measure their success by the number of people who take part. What is being recommended here will very likely reduce uptake. In future, screening programmes should be judged not on uptake but on the quality of informed decision making.'

Several recent articles have shown increasingly conclusive evidence of harm from screening programmes, particularly prostate and breast cancer. Many agencies are calling for more screening, including for disorders such as dementia, but these should similarly be resisted until there is much clearer evidence of benefit. At last the main body of the medical profession is waking up to this shameful state of affairs.

This leads into the increasing tendency to overdiagnosis, and the creation of pseudo-disease. Medicine's ability to diagnose is outpacing our understanding of prognosis, such as finding small tumours, aneurysms and multiple ill-defined risk factors for disease. The trouble is that not all tumours grow, most aneurysms do not burst and most risk factors only occasionally lead to illness. As an editorial in the BMJ (British Medical Journal) of September 2018 says:

Ironically, even though it causes harm, the effects of overdiagnosis look like benefits. People with disease that is overdiagnosed do well because, by definition, their disease was non-progressive. They are 'cured' when the cure was not necessary in the first place. This creates a cycle that reinforces efforts leading to more overdiagnosis.

A screening test that results in substantial overdiagnosis improves survival statistics by diluting the diagnosed pool with many non-progressive cases, which makes screening seem more effective than it is. The spurious rise in incidence makes the case for screening more compelling, thus heightening people's sense of risk – a phenomenon known as the popularity paradox.

The ethics of the doctor's agenda is a complex area that has received too little attention in the past. Again, it relates to the implicit contract between doctor and patient, and the difficulties are most easily highlighted by a discussion of lifestyle advice and screening. Many doctors believe that the right to give unsolicited health and lifestyle advice is inherent in the nature of the relationship. The principle of beneficence comes into play; if the advice is for the patient's good it is ethically justified. Doctors who adhere strongly to such beliefs will view it as unethical to withhold such advice. Some physicians who place patient autonomy high on their list of priorities will seldom offer such advice. To quote Iona Heath, an eminent GP who worked in Kentish Town like me, and one-time president of the RCGP:

Medical science has valued the simple statistics of longevity above any measures of the quality of life. Many of our patients' palpable lack of enthusiasm for the 'lifestyle advice' we are obliged to deliver tells a different story, but the reordering of priorities is nonetheless both insidious and pernicious.... Much more work needs to be done to analyse and describe the limitations of biomedical science, the importance of death, and the overwhelming need to incorporate the patients' own values and aspirations into a system of care which is increasingly driven by standardised protocols. We must recognise the tendency for medical science to become totalitarian.

The insidious nature of this advice has been described as coercive healthism. The medical profession can easily slip into the role of the main arbiter of what is good for people, creating a climate of unjustified fear in an otherwise extremely healthy society. This (probably unstoppable) development is a major barrier to personal autonomy. It is of course a continuation of the old beneficent paternalism, with the further danger of the doctor making negative value judgements when a conflict of health interests arises. This has created a blaming culture, when doctors perceive that patients could do more to help themselves. Smoking and obesity often arouse strong victim-blaming reactions in doctors, and the widespread rise in alcoholism and drug abuse has fuelled this difficulty. These behaviours in patients, and developing the autonomy of the individual, pose major ethical problems for caring doctors; more so in organisations such as the NHS and social care, where resources are clearly finite.

Achieving a balance between beneficence, autonomy and justice is difficult. The communication imperative for the doctor should still be one of understanding and empathy. Issues of fairness, rationing and justice are better left outside the consulting room if at all possible, although this is increasingly difficult as rationing becomes much more overt due to the squeeze on public finances and the constrained budgets of the NHS. Hard choices are having to be made in both local and national health economies, and these intrude more and more into conversations with patients.

One of the difficulties is that the doctor's agenda is being constantly expanded, with uncertain consequences for patients. The cholesterol debate illustrates this increasing nightmare, specifically when looking at the issue of primary prevention of cardiovascular disease. At the time of writing, the QRISK2 and 3 models are the most commonly used cardiovascular risk scoring algorithms for primary prevention. The NICE Cardiovascular disease guideline 2014 (CG181) suggests that clinicians should offer statin medication:

.... for the primary prevention of CVD to people who have a 10% or greater 10-year risk of developing CVD.

This instantly medicalises an awfully large proportion of middle-aged and older adults, who are advised that they should take cholesterol-lowering drugs for the rest of their lives. Apart from the horrendous cost to the Exchequer, this means that most of the adult population will become patients.

Hypertension has now reached plague proportions. This is not a benign diagnosis. Irrespective of treatment, the diagnosis is associated with an increase in absenteeism, sport is avoided, impotence rates quadruple and the 'hypertensive' person now sees himself or herself differently. This is a label that makes people sick, so doctors have to do an awful lot of good to make up for it. David Misselbrook, in his excellent book *Thinking about Patients* (2001), suggests that all hypertensive patients be asked three questions:

1. Do you ever wonder if you might be experiencing side effects from your medication?
2. Do you often think about your blood pressure?
3. Does your blood pressure cause you any problems in your day-to-day life?

He found very high levels of anxiety and a feeling of being stigmatised by the label.

The communication of risk–benefit advice is an interesting area. This is communication at its most difficult, and in this age of evidence-based choice, doctors will need to learn to do it well. As previously alluded to, patients who are well informed, will often make choices of which doctors may not approve. The medical benefits of stroke prevention by warfarin in atrial fibrillation seem to be clear, but in a group of patients who were well informed of the risks and benefits, a significant proportion decided not to choose the intervention (Clarkesmith et al.). Several studies have demonstrated that the method of communicating risk significantly affects patient uptake. Numbers needed to treat patients with mild hypertension to prevent one event provide a very different perspective to saying that taking a particular intervention halves an already small risk. This is an area where 'framing' the questions can easily distort the truth, whatever that is; 'spin' is a more popular word for the same idea.

For example, most doctors are likely to tell patients that trials show that treatment is indicated for mild hypertension, and that treatment will prevent them from having a stroke. They will not usually say that there is a 99.8% probability that treatment will do the individual no good in any given year, that treatment fails to prevent the majority of strokes and that the very marginal benefits of treatment need to be set against the anxiety, medicalisation, side effects and expense of treatment.

The truth is that patients need a certain understanding of basic statistics to understand even the simple medical messages. Sadly, our educational system does not seem to be up to this task and our popular media is worse, so very few patients have any real grasp of the issues at stake. The major problem with risk is the differing frames of reference used by patients and doctors. Doctors use mathematical concepts, absolute risk, relative risk and numbers needed to treat. Patients with varying loci of control see themselves, for very unmathematical reasons, as being high, medium or low risk, and then use the lottery logic of luck, fate and destiny to make an individual and unique assessment. If allowed, patients will tell compelling stories to communicate their perceptions, having already swapped stories in the pub to construct their own sense of reality. Doctors, on the other hand, relate statistics without the persuasive reality and impact of the stories that patients relate. It means that doctors could do worse than learn to relate counter-stories to combat our patients' tales; this is high-level communication and is likely to be unusual. The burning, unanswerable question that patients wants to ask is 'do you really think that taking this tablet for the next 30 years is definitely going to do me more good than harm?'

When trying to achieve shared decision-making, it is permissible, perhaps even morally obligatory, for a doctor to attempt by negotiation, to change the mind of a patient who is making an apparently silly or irrational choice. It is through these genuine negotiations that the doctor and the patient can come to a truly shared understanding of the issues, in a way that is best suited to maximising the values of both parties. Although the decision-making process is shared, the final decision is that of the patient. However, it has to be said that it must be correct, in extreme cases of conflict of belief, for doctors to retain the power not to treat patients if the management choice and plan require them to act in a manner that they believe is unethical. By its very nature, negotiating with a patient may result in an outcome doctors are unsatisfied with. While patients cannot demand a prescription for something the doctor believes to be wholly inappropriate, there is usually a much greyer area where the doctor is persuaded to increase a dose or prescribe something which just might help, but does not honestly believe in its efficacy. The ethics of this, not to mention the view of the GMC and NICE, are debatable. Effective communication in this instance may have been achieved, but at what cost?

Where does all this leave us? It has always seemed to me that one of the ethical hallmarks of good medical communication is a requirement for honesty. There is an imperative for the doctor to seek and confirm understanding in four main areas:

- that the patient is aware that they are an active part of the decision-making process;
- that they are aware of the choices;
- that they are aware of the implications of those choices and;
- that they have assimilated enough specific information on the risks and benefits to allow them to make an informed choice.

A good model must be one of mutual persuasion by two experts, one on medical matters and the other on their own mind and body. This implies that doctors must be prepared to allow themselves to be persuaded by their patients away from their first or second choices of action if the patient's argument is effective, convincing and, most importantly, informed. Doctors often don't like this.

Patients' and doctors' perceptions of patients' problems differ from those expressed both before and after their consultations. Their perceptions about the consultation itself also differ. It has been a long hard lesson, but I now know that asking questions only got me answers. This is one of the problems with traditional history taking; a method of putting communication into a straitjacket to maximise pattern recognition. Doctors are likely to consistently overestimate their patients' understanding, even with the help of Dr Google.

I tried, but the truth is doctors rarely talk to patients about the consequences of their illnesses. We usually do explain a little, but we rarely ask what our patients think, and we also very rarely check whether our patients understand. Sharing any type of management is still unusual. Our consultations are still very one-sided. To communicate effectively the patient's agenda must be searched for and reconciled with the doctors. This is a skilful process, and I have had a lot of practice. My desired outcome was a shared understanding and a shared management plan, but I achieved it much less often than I would have liked.

My attitudes are what governed my behaviour. I would just like to point out that most conventional educational theory implies, and in some cases even states, that knowledge governs behaviour. Health educators are driven unceasingly (and often fruitlessly) by this belief. I am not saying that knowledge does not change behaviour, but it only works when what is learned changes an attitude about, say, a procedure, a screening opportunity or a loosely held belief (e.g. for or against the legalisation of cannabis). This, of course, makes the point that not all attitudes are equal; some are much more entrenched than others, and much less amenable to the voice of reason. Attitudes do change, even mine, but usually slowly. If I started again, I would concentrate more on finding out the attitudes of my patients to the slings and arrows of outrageous medicine, and might be more effective in steering them towards doing what is currently thought to be good for them.

Of course, the same applies to me, I have attitudes, too. When my attitudes clashed with those of my patients, 'professionalism' was the fall-back position, followed by a strong cup of coffee and a gripe to my partners.

It is now well-known that patients have a cycle of readiness to change. This was first described in relation to changing smoking behaviours in the early 1980s, but it is now clear that patients often must go through several unhelpful challenges to their health beliefs before achieving the necessary will to accept treatment. Often a sort of epiphany is needed that allows patients to take autonomous control of their illness. Doctors must ask themselves; do I really want to involve my patients? If not, why not? The simple answer is that most of the profession still do not regard patient-centred, evidence-based, shared decision-making as worth the time and emotional effort. And if they feel like that, all the knowledgeable and clever teaching in the world is going to make very little, if any, difference. In fact, most humans do not need much teaching in communication. In my personal experience, many young registrars have become really 'good' communicators almost overnight in the sense of involving their patients, following a real attitude change brought about by an overbearing trainer, or a realisation of the annoying consequences of failing the impending postgraduate examination. Of course, they can then improve and practise the skills until they become automatic and instinctive, but the first and fundamental step is the change in attitude. Get the attitude right by thinking, then let instinct, experience and evolution take over and the results can be almost magical.

I believe the most important factor in deciding whether a therapeutic relationship is likely to be effective is the attitude of both parties. If the doctor intrinsically disapproves of the patient's behaviour, the relationship is unlikely to succeed. The most effective relationship appears, not surprisingly, to be a trusting one; for trust to develop, the patient must believe the doctor is on their side. The other thing about trust is that it takes time to build up. As a rule of thumb, the more they see you the more they trust you.

Doctors have a difficult task, and from time to time we need to take a long, hard, honest look at our own prejudices. Today there are a multitude of gender, sexual and religious views that individual doctors are faced with. These may clash with their own religious, ethnic and societal beliefs. Perhaps all young doctors thinking of working with patients who have very different views must, early in their careers, take time to look critically at their own attitudes to these patients. If they find themselves seriously wanting, then maybe a career in pathology beckons?

I know more about the way I think after reading Daniel Kahneman's *Thinking, Fast and Slow*. I realise I am programmed to jump to conclusions and then to look for facts that will confirm them, my *confirmation bias*. Patients are no better; in a conversation with me, patients hear messages that I may or may not have meant, but in the subsequent dialogue, and after leaving the consultation, they will continue to search for evidence that confirms their initial conclusion. This 'seeking data that is compatible with the beliefs we already hold' is, of course, the opposite of testing hypotheses by trying to refute them, which is what science tells us is the only reliable approach.

And of the future? I quote my co-author of eighth edition of *The Doctor's Communication Handbook*, Francesca Frame, a Cambridge GP:

Healthcare risks being reduced to a transactional arrangement; a transfer of information, the provision of tests and medications. As doctors, we know that it is so much more than this. The art of a consultation is to reach a shared understanding of the patient's concern in order for the consultation be truly effective. This complex and nuanced process is often therapeutic in itself, something that is little understood or acknowledged by the public. Digital solutions cannot replicate this yet. Patients will not know what they are missing out on, but we shall.

We are also well-aware of the risk of over-medicalisation and the long-term harm that this can cause. We do not yet know what the impact of having a doctor or AI-substitute just a tap away on every smartphone does to the public's perception of their health, and their perceived need to access healthcare, although I have my own suspicions. We must protect patients from potential harms of easier and faster ways to access healthcare until they are proven to be effective; convenience does not equate to better. The risks may not be obvious to our patients, but they are obvious to us.

I will finish with an old quote: The crucial paradox is that in the consultation the doctor makes the treatment decisions; after the consultation, decision-making lies with the patient.

This book was written by Royal Command. In 2008 I was awarded the MBE and when being given the award by the Queen herself, she asked why I thought it had been given to me? I told her that I thought it was for writing books to improve communication between doctors and patients. Holding my hand, she looked deep into my eyes and said enthusiastically, 'Now that is very important, I do hope you carry on'. Then while trying to walk backwards and turn at the same time I tripped over. Hey ho.

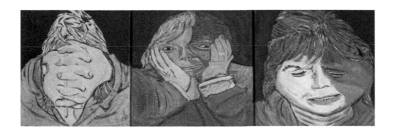

ICE Version 2 Acrylic on canvas by PT, 2010.

REFERENCES

Brodersen J et al. 2018. Focusing on overdiagnosis as a driver of too much medicine. *BMJ* 362, k3494.

Clarkesmith DE, Pattison, HM, Lip, GY, & Lane DA. 2013. Educational intervention improves anticoagulation control in atrial fibrillation patients: The TREAT randomised trial. *PLOS ONE* 8(9), e74037.

Eysenck HJ et al. 1960. Smoking and personality. *Br Med J* 1(5184), 1456–1460.

Eysenck HJ. 1964. Personality and cigarette smoking. *Life Sci* 3(7), 77–792.

Eysenck HJ. 1988. The respective importance of personality, cigarette smoking and interaction effects for the genesis of cancer and coronary heart disease. *Per Individ Differe* 9(2), 453–464.

Godlee F. 2019. Cancer screening: From uptake to informed decision making. *BMJ* 367, l5931.

Heath I. 1999. William Pickles Lecture 1999: 'Uncertain clarity': Contradiction, meaning, and hope. *Br J Gen Pract* 49(445), 651–7.

Kahneman D. 2011. *Thinking, Fast and Slow.* New York: Farrar, Straus and Giroux.

"Salgo v. Leland Stanford Etc. Bd. Trustees, 317 P.2d 170, 154 Cal. App. 2d 560 – CourtListener.com". CourtListener.

Smith SK, Trevena L, Simpson JM et al. 2010. A decision aid to support informed choices about bowel cancer screening among adults with low education: Randomised controlled trial. *BMJ* 341, c5370.

Stimson GV & Webb B. 1975. *Going to See the Doctor.* London: Routledge & Keegan Pail.

Appendix

CHAPTER 3

Very early on we linked up with the Manchester-based Group, North West Spanner, led by Penny Morris with Ernest Dalton and several others, who had been working occasionally in Professor David Metcalfe's Department of General Practice in Manchester (He had replaced Pat Byrne). Peter H and Theo used this brilliant group of actors for many years on their regular consultation courses.

Spanner was for real, their theatre group first performed in the 1970s as part of the 'agitprop' theatre movement. Their plays were not only commenting on industrial and political unrest but also seeking to encourage it! These plays were performed in factories and working men's clubs across the country, exploring the relationships and pressures of the factory floor and looking at the debates taking place every day. The Spanner plays are perhaps best summed up by the reaction of a Tory councillor, who in 1977 tried to destroy the Spanner theatre group by cutting their funding and claiming their plays called for 'blood on the streets'. They were brilliant at playing patients and could give doctors very accurate feedback on how effective their consulting skills really were. The rules were often crucial. Overconfident doctors being quietly but firmly shown that their patient's view was some distance from their own.

DOCTORS' STYLE: PETER TATE, SEPTEMBER 1980

This was my first venture into medical writing.

I have to be honest here, I never met Pat Byrne, once saw him across a room at a meeting with John Horder who was a close friend, but never actually spoke to him. Years later I did become friends with his co-researcher Barry Long, a tall booming Welshman, who reckoned he had done all the work anyway. In 1991 we were at a course together, here he was all six feet four inch of him, bluff, gruff and great value. He then taught health-care management to anyone that would listen and was based at Swansea University. He told me a story of going to Bart's in 1990 to apply for a post directing a study into doctor–patient communication. A serious little man interviewed him, saying that it was a coincidence having the same name as a famous but long dead researcher in the same field. Barry, tapping his chest, insisted it was he, but the interviewer jovially poopoo'd him saying the research was classical and far too long ago, he, the Barry in point, was unquestionably dead, which leads inescapably to the John Wayne line 'The Hell I am!' He did not get the job.

Pat Byrne had just retired when sadly in late February 1980 he dropped dead. David, knowing my hero worship, asked me to write his chapter.

I append a considerably edited version, retaining the headings[1]:

Doctor's Style by Peter Tate

A doctor's style is an amalgam of behaviours derived from his personal beliefs, knowledge, experience and skilfulness. The individual variations are infinite but certain broad categories are recognisable. Most doctors practice towards the doctor-centred end of a spectrum, which is the traditional authoritarian approach based on the assumption that the doctor is responsible for his patient's health and will go through his agenda for the patient. At the other end of the scale, the doctor is seen as much less authoritarian, the responsibility for health is shared and the patient is encouraged to go through his own agenda not the doctor's.

1. REASONS FOR ADOPTING A STYLE
   Most doctors have never been trained to consult in a general practice setting.
   A doctor's attitudes are clearly reflected in the way he deals with patients, but these attitudes are also related to his skilfulness.

2. FLEXIBILITY OF STYLE
   There is evidence that when doctors have developed a set of behaviours, they use these stock patterns again and again and that many of these behaviours are not significantly influenced by the patient's presenting problem. No doctors appear to span the whole range; those described as patient-centred showed more flexibility, but the overall results show a chastening rigidity.

3. STYLE RELATED TO AUTHORITY

Each individual doctor's need for power is probably one of the main guiding factors in the manner in which he practices medicine.

The traditional authoritarian approach is adopted by the majority of doctors. The sharing and listening approach probably decreases some of the doctor's authority. Doctors who wish to have a lot of influence over their patients may thus consciously or unconsciously maintain a degree of uncertainty.

As he is seen as a healer a doctor's words have the power to reduce anxiety and reassure, even if the scientific content of the message is suspect.

4. SEATING POSITION

Doctors who sit behind their desk maintain a rigid distance between themselves and their patients. Every business executive is aware of the maintaining of power differentials by this method.

The absence of a desk will normally reduce the perceived authority of the doctor unless he compensates in some other way, such as wearing a white coat.

5. DRESS

6. INFORMATION GATHERING

The first phase of any consultation is usually concerned with the doctor gathering information.

It seems that most doctors develop stock openings consisting of both verbal and non-verbal behaviours, repeated time and again. In general practice usually because a working hypothesis has been made very early in the consultation. When using this method of gathering information, it is usually the presenting complaint that is fixed on, the implication being that the doctor is looking for answers that will enable him to solve that problem for the patient.

Often the doctor returns to questioning again and again until almost the end. The doctor who only follows the path of the presenting remarks is very likely to miss any other reasons for attendance, producing a higher proportion of what has been termed dysfunctional consultations.

7. INFORMATION GIVING

One definition of information is 'that which reduces uncertainty' and, as discussed previously, maintaining uncertainty can be a method of maintaining influence. Doctors who habitually give little or cryptic information to their patients are consciously or unconsciously maintaining power over them.

There is considerable evidence on the relatively poor uptake of medical advice and it is very probable that changes in style could improve this. It may become a matter of style.

8. PRESCRIBING

The therapeutic art of prescribing is still expected by most patients and their doctors, despite orchestrated campaigns designed to lessen these expectations.

9. TIME

When doctors discuss the reason for their behaviours, the commonest factor mentioned is one of time.

10. IMPLICATIONS FOR TRAINING

Teaching doctors how to consult, as well as teaching them clinical medicine, has only recently become fashionable again, most obviously in the fields of psychiatry and general practice.

11. SUMMARY

Individual doctors vary in their style of consulting. His style is a unique blend of behaviours determined by his skills and his attitudes, and influenced by his personality, experience and education.

All doctors should be aware of the effects of their ways of behaving on their patients. Most importantly, we should learn that these behaviours are not immutable. We can all, with (a little) help (from our friends), learn new behaviours and skills, possibly bringing about changes in our attitudes. Future training of all doctors must be intimately concerned with the question of style.

THE FIRST APPEARANCE OF 'CYCLES OF CARE'

Paper presented at the annual conference of the British Psychological Society, Aberdeen, 1980. Research and training in the skills of communication between general practitioner and patient, David Pendleton and Peter Tate.

ABSTRACT

This paper will outline a major problem in doctor–patient communication, the problem of compliance. Secondly, it will suggest a model to locate research in the field of communication between GP and patient. Thirdly, it will present a brief outline of research of this kind underway at Oxford. Finally, it will describe GP training in the Oxford region and will show how the findings of the basic research are being applied in the vocational training of GPs.

<u>Alternative models of the effect of other variables on compliance with</u>

<u>medical advice</u>

Model 1 : Direct

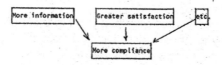

Model 2 : Mediation

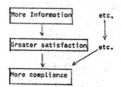

<u>Input, process and outcomes in primary medical care</u>

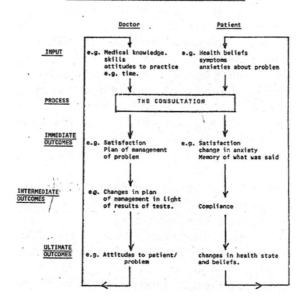

Here is a take from a magazine of that time, 1981.

'An Oxford psychologist's research with a surgery video suggests that probing deeper does not waste a GP's time. Psychologist David Pendleton and GP Dr Peter Tate: 'Until you understand the patient's own theory about his problem, you can't begin to treat him properly'.

When that dread-inspiring lady Mrs Bloggs walks through the surgery door, plonks herself down with an air of permanence and begins a blow-by-blow account of her own diagnosis, how do you react?

Do you let her ramble on while you flip through the notes? Do you gently cut her short? Do you take the upper hand: 'Just say where it hurts', you ask Bloggs, 'I'll say what's wrong with you'.

Or do you listen, with growing amazement, to the full saga of Mrs Bloggs's startling concept of her own insides?

It is a question which has preoccupied Oxford University psychologist David Pendleton and his video machine for the last three years.

A research academic, Dr Pendleton – with the help of four local GPs and the Royal College – has been studying the vexed but intriguing question of doctor–patient communication.

And one of the central conclusions he has reached is that GPs do not take enough trouble to find out what their patients think of their own bodies.

'You've got to encourage both parties – GP and patient to volunteer more to each other'.

One of the family doctors helping the psychologist with his research is Abingdon GP and training course organiser Dr Peter Tate.

For the past three years, with the patients' consent, he has videotaped his own consultations at Abingdon Health Centre, played them back and tried to apply the theory to the facts.

As a result, he is an enthusiastic partisan of Dr Pendleton's 'ask-the-patient' views despite the apparent drawbacks, such as increased consultation time.

'Nobody goes to the doctor with just a sore throat. They go with an idea about that symptom. Most doctors overlook this', he says.

'But until you understand the patient's own theory about his problem, you won't understand why the patient has come to see you, and you can't begin to treat him properly'.

A beautiful example had occurred in the previous day's surgery. An American had turned up wanting help with losing weight. Straightforward dietary advice?

Dr Pendleton approvingly takes up the story. What Pete did was take a little time and ask: 'Why do you want to lose weight?'

Out, slowly, came the story that his brother, of similar age and build, had just had a heart attack. Because Pete took the trouble to find out the patient's own theories, he uncovered another problem – anxiety.

'Any doctor worth his salt would have considered the possibility of heart disease. But how many would have brought it into the open? The patient was left reassured'.

Dr Pendleton's research has now been enshrined in the training offered to young GPs in several Oxfordshire teaching practices.

It is based on the principle that a successful consultation is not one conducted to any particular formula, but one in which a number of 'tasks' have been achieved.

At the heart of the training is a 12-point 'consultation tasks rating scale' which trainees use to assess their own performances on videotape.

The trainees check-off on the scale how well they think they have dealt with the nature and aetiology of each problem; nothing unusual in that. But the scale then goes on to such Pendeltonian subjects as what the patient thinks about his illness, and what effect this has on him physically, psychologically and socially.

Dr Tate does not agree that probing that little bit deeper necessarily leads to longer consultations. Research shows, says Dr Pendleton, that the more questions a doctor asks the fewer a patient does, so it evens out.

The practical benefits are enormous for both doctor and patient in terms of satisfaction, compliance and national health.

'It will satisfy the patient and leave him better equipped to handle his own health problems in the future'.

One possibility is that doctor and patient will become so empathetic that the patient keeps on going back to the surgery for sheer visit satisfaction.

But Dr Tate has no reservations. 'Before the videos, I wasn't finding out why patients were coming to see me. I wasn't going that step further. Now I've learnt ... not to listen ... but to hear what the patient is telling me'.

David and I were invited to present the group's ideas to an Anglo/French collaboration in late 1981. We were assured that it would be bilingual, they fibbed, we were the only Anglos. The conference was in an old monastery just outside Aix. The colours were autumnal gold and my abiding memory is of the sweet all-pervasive smell of Gauloise cigarettes, with ashtrays piled high to overflowing by the end of the day.

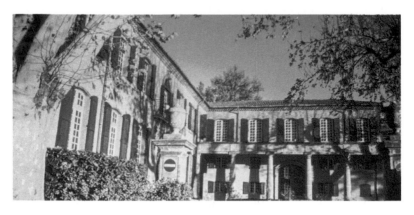

An old monastery outside Aix.

My wife and my two very young children came too, as did Jenny King, and after a pleasant if incomprehensible week we got to Nice Airport to be greeted by a sign that read: Heathrow Annul Neige. We got a plane to the then new Charles de Gaulle airport in Paris but could get no further for two days as London remained snowbound. We stayed in as yet not officially opened accommodation and were reduced to using Le Monde as a temporary nappy substitute.

This article, 15th of October 1981, tells how far we had got by then.

Putting consulting on the curriculum

'Although she had only come for a repeat prescription of the Pill, it didn't take much digging from the doctor to find that the new patient was probably pregnant, certainly unmarried and extremely indecisive about what she should do.

The consultation was a model of excellence, replete with open questions, non-judgmental explanations, and encouragement to self-reliance. Together, doctor and patient plotted the immediate future with the patient taking a pregnancy test, finding out if the vital university exam in eight months' time could be postponed and discussing the unforeseen event with her boyfriend.

Later, the doctor, watching her performance on video, weighed up the weaknesses and strengths of the consultation. She had, she thought, succeeded in not making moral judgments. She had felt it was very important not to show her feelings, not to reveal whether she would approve a termination. But she was also dissatisfied. 'I don't think I got her to talk enough. I didn't feel able to counsel her properly', she admitted to a trainer and group of fellow-trainees who had been watching the consultation, each with pen poised over a consultation rating scale. For the patient was a student at Oxford's Department of Experimental Psychology, acting as a volunteer guinea pig at a weekend at Cumberland Lodge, Windsor, Surrey for trainees to learn how to assess their consultation skills and their ability to perform a set list of consultation tasks. The course, which is organised regionally and backed up by district and surgery training is unique to Oxford. Indeed, it is still being developed. Taking as its baseline the fact that patients complain about how GPs communicate more than anything else, and that a half of medical advice is ignored, and a half of prescribed medicines are not taken, the course is aimed at answering the question: 'Can we teach the art of consultation?' and exploits to the full the recent developments in video technology. The concept of teaching trainees how to communicate with their patients resulted from a collaboration between general practice and social psychology and began by a happy accident four years ago.

When David Pendleton was accepted at Oxford University to study for a DPhil, he decided to look at communication in medicine. Formerly a polytechnic lecturer in Leeds, he had been studying how teachers could communicate better with parents, head teachers, educational psychologists and the like. He approached a university doctor, to see if it might be possible to get inside a GP's surgery and was directed to Dr John Hasler, Oxford's regional organiser in vocational training and honorary secretary of the Royal College of General Practitioners. Since then, Pendleton says, his feet have hardly touched the ground. In four years, he has videoed 2,500 consultations, analysing in detail 84 of them, and, with three trainers, he has studied some 350 academic papers on communication from the fields of medicine and psychology.

To begin with, Pendleton, with Dr Hasler, and Dr Peter Tate – who took a six-month sabbatical to help Pendleton – were concerned with the relatively conventional task of drawing up lists of behavioural skills that might aid a doctor in the surgery.

A good deal of work had already been carried out in this area, particularly by the late Professor Pat Byrne, who analysed 2,000 tapes of consultations and came up with a list of useful skills, such as standing to greet the patient, asking open questions – 'How do you feel?' – rather than closed ones – as 'Have you got a headache?' – and in making a consultation patient-centred rather than doctor-centred. But teaching behavioural skills led to a dead end. 'We could specify a number of skills', explained Pendleton, 'but we constantly kept coming against the question "So what?" If I do all these things, does it mean that I am a better doctor. The answer was that we didn't know'.

It was then the team turned to studying thousands of videoed consultations, working through the literature, to draw up a list of seven 'consultation tasks'.

The first: **To define the reasons why the patient has come today,** may seem obvious but, according to Dr Tate, is something doctors rarely do. At the extreme, this results in 'the dysfunctional consultation', where the doctor and patient are talking at cross purposes. But doctors rarely seek the patient's views on why he has come, what his concerns and expectations are and what are the effects of his problem.

This is true, he says, of the second task: **To consider other problems**. In only 2% of consultations do doctors consider risk factors and the patient's background. We make great play of being 'the family doctor', yet most doctors know little about the patient's family, Dr Tate said.

The third task: **To choose an appropriate action for each problem**, underlines the fact that patients bring, on average three and a half problems to the doctor's surgery.

The fourth: **To share the doctor's understanding, of the problems with each patient**, takes account of a major finding of Pendleton's research – that doctors experience more communication problems with working class patients and, as a consequence, volunteer fewer explanations.

The fifth: **To involve the patient in the management and encourage him to accept appropriate responsibility**.

The sixth: **To use time and resources appropriately**, takes account of GP's need to perform all these tasks in an average of six and a half minutes.

The seventh: **To establish and maintain a relationship with the patient which facilitates the achievement of the above tasks,** emphasises the team's belief that influence of the GP consultation can be spread over repeated meetings.

What is obvious about this analysis of general practice is the debt it owes to video. And video as a teaching aid cannot be underestimated. One of the trainers said his family's table manners had improved dramatically as a result videotaping Sunday lunch.

It is one thing to hand over a tasks list, to tell trainees about doctor-centred and patient-centred consulting and warn of the dangers of dysfunctional consultations. It is another to present them with real-life examples which can be discussed and analysed at leisure, as the Oxford trainees were able to do at the training weekend at Cumberland Lodge.

First the trainees heard Dr Tate explain the philosophy behind the task list. They were told of the difference between doctor-centred consulting (where the doctor is in charge, takes the decisions for the patient, asks closed questions, looks for patterns, wears a white coat and sits behind a desk) and the patient-centred consultation (where the doctor allows the patient to work through his own agenda, asks exploratory questions, and encourages the patient to put forward his own ideas, gives the patient more responsibility and has less 'healing powers'). Neither model is right or wrong, said Dr Tate. Both are appropriate at different times. But it has been discovered that doctors can rarely move freely between the two models, and training is aimed at giving trainees this kind of flexibility. Then came the video examples. The trainees watched doctors being doctor-centred and patient-centred; they saw an example of a dysfunctional consultation where the doctor guessed at the illness that had recently taken a patient to hospital and was wrong; they saw a 'sheep in wolf's clothing', where the doctor rapped out questions to the patient like a general to a private, yet somehow allowed the patient total control over the consultation; they saw a 'wolf in sheep's clothing', where the doctor's honeyed exclamations of sympathy prevented the patient from getting a word in edgeways.

The trainees were bursting with indignation, ready to rip some of the unfortunate participants apart. But it was quickly made clear that this was not the name of the game. Rules for observing videotaped consultations, from 'brutal experience' insist that the discussion must begin with what is seen to be good, moving slowly to areas of disagreement. 'This is a building, not a demolition exercise'.

The rules, Dr Tate explained, underline that what is being offered is different to the conventional hospital–orientated education. 'In hospital students are taught by destructive comment, by fear and insult on the ward round'.

Also important is the team's conviction that the aim of the course is not to produce 'chocolate doctors who all come out the same'. 'We are not out to destroy doctors' idiosyncrasies. We want to build on the best abilities and improve on the weak points. The important thing is what they achieve – how they achieve it doesn't matter a hoot'.

In the afternoon session at Cumberland Lodge, the trainees role-played, and all were incisive, observant and helpful and kind to the surrogate patients who included, as well as the pregnant student, an anxious Valium-dependent, alcoholic salesman and a career girl who, having moved into a remote cottage, where she was totally dependent on her car, discovered she was a grand mal epileptic.

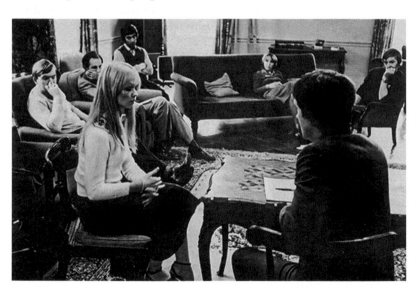

Trainees role-play at Cumberland Lodge.

Nobody was reduced to tears, nobody felt threatened or embarrassed. After all, with less than two months' experience of general practice behind them, what reputation did any of them have to lose?

The value of the rules will be seen in the 'back-up' courses where trainees' real consultations are videoed and discussed. Such rules will be indispensable if plans go ahead to use video and the assessment system as a tool of peer audit for established GPs, and, as is now under serious consideration by the RCGP Board of Examiners, as an alternative to the College membership exam.

And the trainees' reactions? On the whole they enjoyed the exercise, whilst maintaining a healthy scepticism. Some said they feared that improving consultation skills could lead them to manipulate patients or to interfere too much in a patient's problems. Another trainee said he thought trainers assumed that trainees, coming directly from eight years in hospital, had no clinical problems – whereas, rather than concentrating on communicating with patients, he would have preferred a bit more on GP clinical care. So far, Oxford has not proved that training doctors to communicate with patients produces better outcomes. 'Give us a couple of years for that', said Dr Hasler. David Pendleton points out that in only 20% of consultations does the GP actually cure the patient. In the other 80%, doctors deal with the chronically ill, with self-limiting illness and with patients who come, not with a problem, but with their fears that they might have a problem.

'Of course, clinical skills are important. But we think that a successful outcome is the result of successful clinical medicine and successful communication. Curing someone without communicating with them does not necessarily result in a satisfied patient'.

Mr Pendleton, together with Dr Hasler, is now working on the first draft of a core curriculum for GP trainees which will aim to reduce the diversity of subjects that trainers randomly pick to teach their trainees. Consultation skills are certain to be a major priority in the curriculum which is likely to be backed by the RCGP. The result will probably be that the Oxford cross fertilization between medicine and psychology could have a profound influence on the way general practice is taught in the future'.

This article also emphasises how necessary the use of actors were in teaching the consultation.

Reference

1. *Doctor–Patient Communication*: Eds. Pendleton and Hasler. Academic Press, 1983. ISBN 0-12-549880-2 75–85.

CHAPTER 4

I attach here the essay I wrote in December 1986 at the end of my American sojourn. It is unedited, exactly as written then.

Should Patients Take More Responsibity for Their Own Medical Management?

December 1986, Peter Tate

Why should patients wish for more responsibility? What is it they have to gain? Greater autonomy perhaps, greater control over their own destiny? More important perhaps is with increasing responsibility the greater the likelihood of following an agreed therapeutic course leading to a better outcome. Increased patient involvement can undoubtedly improve the effectiveness of medical intervention. This is of course a doctor's argument. John Stuart Mill the famous libertarian, put the patient's argument quite succinctly as far back as 1859. 'Over himself, his own body and mind the individual is sovereign'.[1]

In fact, the history of medicine over the last 2,000 years is very definitely weighted against patients taking much responsibility for their own health. Hippocrates advised doctors to conceal any important prognostic information from their patients[2] and Plato stated quite categorically that physicians had a right to employ lies for good and noble purposes. The Greeks laid the foundation of the ethic which has lasted to this day that good physicians should, not could, be authoritarian, manipulative and even frankly, deceitful. This stance was entrenched in quite the best of motives, helping sick people required those who were ill to respect and value medical authority because without this there could be no cure. Participation by the sick person in any decision making was seen as counterproductive, an activity to be discouraged. Doctor knows best was undoubtedly good for you. The trouble with this pragmatic view is ultimately the lack of respect given to people when they are ill. This respect seems to have two necessary dimensions, concern for patients' welfare and respect for their wishes. In the Greek ethic the first element was there but not the second.

In 1956, Szasz and Hollender set out three basic models of the physician–patient relationship.

- Activity–passivity
- Guidance–cooperation
- Mutual participation

The third model was still seen to be very unusual. Only a year later came the first use of the term, 'informed consent' in a Californian Appeal Court. In 1972, Robert Veatch described three idealised 'models for ethical medicine in a revolutionary age'. In his first model the doctor is the cool calculating scientist dealing only with facts, his role is to present all those facts to his patient and let the patient make up her mind and then carry out those wishes. There is no moral stance and no emotional involvement. Patient decision making has appeared with a vengeance, doctor paternalism has gone, but at what cost? The caritas, all the good inherent in the old Greek ethic, the concern for the patient's welfare, the traditional physician beneficence, has gone. This is your modern doctor plumber.

In this second model the doctor assumes the priestly mantle. The patient has 'sinned' by getting sick. The decision making has reverted to the doctor and the time honoured trap for all patients who do not follow doctors' orders is there, the addition of another 'sin'. This is naked paternalism and the easiest way to spot this model in action is to recognise the speaking as a doctor syndrome. 'Speaking as your doctor I feel it is definitely time you underwent surgical sterilisation'.

The decision here is in fact a moral not a medical one but the priest doctor is presumed to have competence in both areas by virtue of his medical degree.

The third idealised model was the best of the bunch. He called it the 'contractual model'. He envisaged the contract between doctor and patient as a non-legalistic statement of general obligations and benefits to both parties. The doctor acknowledges that the patient ought to have control over his or her own life whenever significant decisions are to be made. Reciprocally the patient recognises that the doctor has the requisite skill to make necessary technical decisions helpful to achieving the goal that the patient has agreed to. This of course means that important value-laden aspects are dealt with first and this whole covenant calls for a sharing of the decision-making responsibility. This model also implies that patients would expect their doctors to take no major action without allowing them, the patients, to make the necessary decisions but they would not expect to be consulted on all the technical details. It also implies that doctors retain the right not to enter into the contract or to force them to perform acts morally abhorrent to them.

Howard Brody in his book *Ethical Decisions in Medicine*[5] accepts this model as the best single statement of the ideal doctor–patient relationship and as a result he states that it is imperative for the doctor to tell his patient the truth about her condition in a language she can understand unless the doctor has an overwhelming reason to believe that a degree of harm, more serious than merely temporary emotional depression would follow as a result.

In their book, *Clinical Ethics*, Jonsen, Siegler and Winslade[6] take a deep breath and come out with an ethical rank order of the factors that should influence medical decision making.

They are top of the list, patient preferences, second the medical indications, third the quality of life and last socioeconomic factors.

If Veatch's contractual or covenant model really is the one to aim for this has very major implications in the field of doctor–patient communication.

Tuckett et al. in *Meetings between Experts*, a thorough report on a detailed piece of research about sharing ideas between doctors and patients, found that doctors rarely talked about the consequences of illness and although doctors usually gave a few reasons which might give patients some idea what the doctors thought about their condition the doctors spent little or no time trying to share what patients thought. The consultations in other words were very one-sided. Doctors and patients did not manage to achieve a dialogue and so did not share or exchange ideas to any meaningful degree. In fact, doctors seemed to actively discourage patients from presenting their views. These doctors were UK GP volunteers and the work was carried out within the last seven years.

If patients are to take more responsibility for their own medical management, they need more information than it is usual for them to receive at present. They almost always want as much information as possible, the fact that we doctors often do not accept this is probably one of the most common errors of clinical practice.

Howard Waitzkin in a hard-hitting review attack on doctor–patient communication[8] highlights this fact and revealed that American doctors' performance was similar to that found by Tuckett. He found that doctors spent very little time giving information to their patients, little more than a minute on average in encounters lasting about 20 minutes. In fact, the doctors thought they were doing much better and overestimated the time they spent giving information by about a factor of nine.

Byrne and Long in their classic *Doctors Talking to Patients*[9] analysed in detail the behaviour of doctors in the consultation and found that they could be described along a spectrum ranging from doctor-centred that is those who went through their agenda for patients, patients made little or no contribution except to answer questions, to the other end of the spectrum they called patient-centred. Here doctors took on more and more of the patients' agenda, their ideas concerns, beliefs and values. The doctor-centred style was by far the commonest and is a high control information gathering dominant behaviour designed intrinsically to prevent patients taking too much responsibility for their own health. It is the traditional method of consulting and for many patients is reassuring and anxiety relieving. It is nice to have a powerful doctor take away responsibility for one's illness.

Towards the patient-centred end of the spectrum there is a much greater sharing of understanding and most important a greater sharing of decision making. The far end of this scale, the fully patient-centred doctor, will concentrate wholly on his or her patient's agenda to the exclusion logically of his own. He respects totally the autonomy of his patients, shares decision making, actively searches for their values and beliefs, is non-coercive, a professional reflective counsellor. Non-directive and non-involved. The fully patient-centred doctor on this scale is no paradigm of virtue, he is a cop out, as in the first Veatch model.

The other major contribution made by Byrne and Long to this debate is to reveal that we doctors were what we were. We were not the flexible talented responders we thought we were. They demonstrated conclusively that doctors with a particular style be it patient- or doctor-centred, has a very limited ability to change behaviour with different patients or different situations.

Pendleton et al. in their book *The Consultation: An Approach to Learning and Teaching*[10] proposed a teaching framework for GPs based on the concept of discovering patients' ideas concerns and expectations and then sharing understanding and decision making. This sharing is not fully patient-centred in the Byrne and Long sense, the doctor here has not totally abrogated his responsibility. After all, much of the resentment in the medical profession of criticism of its paternalism is rooted in the belief that responsibility for patients involves strong moral obligations and considerable self-sacrifice. The strategy advocated by Pendleton et al. is centred round tasks for doctors to achieve in a consultation, it is not prescriptive in style but by the advocacy of shared decision making places the doctor more to the centre of Byrne and Long's scale. If GPs consult using the task system advocated in this book, they will share decisions with their patients, this is a major move to increasing patient involvement in their own healthcare.

The essay title, 'Should patients take more responsibility for their own medical management?' begs the question more than what? Patients have always been in a powerful position in relationship to doctors. More than doctors care to admit perhaps and they have exercised this power in many ways. They don't take our advice or our treatments. Podell[11] and many others have demonstrated the miserable uptake of medical advice, approximately one-third is rejected out of hand, one-third taken in such a way as to be ineffective and only one-third taken effectively. Patients also change doctors, need not come to us at all, go to alternative practitioners. In America they can and often do, have a different doctor for each different complaint. It is our role as a profession to help our patients use their power of choice more responsibly by giving people valid criteria on which to make judgements. The consultation is central to this and the tasks strategy advocated by Pendleton et al. seems the most effective model proposed so far.

There is a tremendous burgeoning of patient advice from a myriad of sources matching the ever-increasing consumerism in our society, this advice is not always good or even helpful in allowing people to take more responsibility for their own health. It must be our profession's job to try to influence this consumerism appropriately and effectively for our patients' benefit. King et al. produced a little book for patients titled *Making the Most of Your Doctor*[12] based on the Pendleton et al.'s *Consultation* approach and the RCGP 'What sort of doctor' report[14]. In the book patients were encouraged to get involved in their own healthcare and shown some criteria by which to make judgements on the quality of the healthcare they were receiving and could receive. In the field of general practice, they were encouraged, using check lists, to see how accessible their doctor was, how to make some sort of judgements on clinical competence, how to assess their doctor as a communicator and also to make some assessment of the values important to their doctors. The profession was rather nettled by this book which attempted to educate patients in ways of taking more responsibility for their own management, feeling that some of this increased scrutiny might be unfair, there is always the paranoia of being found wanting and if patients are to take more responsibility doctors will have to come to terms with this. In American literature there are many more books of a similar ilk, some much more radical.

People are becoming more active, less passive in their dealings with doctors, they make choices not subject to control by their doctors. If shared decision making is the goal can patients be given skills to influence their doctors? No patient seeks medical care without some desire to influence their doctor, they want particular medications, sicknotes, life insurance, approval for their illness behaviour. They want their doctors to relieve their pain, ease their worries, get them slim, extend their lives and keep their secrets. They want words spoken or written, some act performed. Can patients improve their ability to influence doctors? Greenfield et al. in a fascinating paper[14] show that they probably can. They coached patients with peptic ulcers on how to ask questions and negotiate in medical decision making, they were even given rehearsals and role-play and those patients so coached did much better than patients in the control group. Their pain was less, their physical activity was more and they were much more satisfied.

If we doctors genuinely wish our patients to take more responsibility it means we must be prepared to share more of ourselves. At a simple level we must be prepared to give information of our services in a clear easily accessible way, practice leaflets are surely a must. But at a deeper level, if we are actively searching out our patients' beliefs and value systems, is it not appropriate for a genuine and un-Machiavellian sharing to allow our patients to see some of our own values and beliefs? The goal of shared decision making alters some of the debates on patient held records, confidentiality and amounts of information shared. If doctors and patients fairly reach a shared decision without undue coercion, the concept of mutual persuasion advocated by Smith is helpful here[15], then these decisions become individual. If a shared decision is reached that the patient should see their record, have a copy of it or whatever then that is fine, the difficult bit is the communication involved in reaching that shared decision.

The title of this essay is misleading. Patients are taking more responsibility for their own medical management, we as a profession must concentrate on the implications this has, particularly in the field of communication. I will leave the final quote of this essay to Jay Katz, the American Ethicist[16].

'Can patients be trusted to participate more fully in the decisions that affect their well-being? The answer one gives to this question will shape the subsequent analysis of all the other problems. I believe patients can be trusted. If anyone were to contest this belief I would ask, 'can physicians be trusted to make decisions for patients?' Both must be trusted but, they can only be trusted if they first learn to trust each other'.

References

1. Mill John Stuart 1859. 1982. *On Liberty*. Franklin Library.
2. W. Jones (Trans.). 1967. *Hippocrates 'Decorum'*. Cambridge Press, 297.
3. Szasz TS & Hollender MH. 1956. A contribution to the philosophy of medicine. The basic models of the doctor–patient relationship. *Arch Intern Med*. 97, 585–592.
4. Veatch RM. Models for ethical medicine in a revolutionary age. *Hastings Cent Rep*. 2(72), 5.
5. Brody H. 1976. *Ethical Decisions in Medicine*. Boston: Little Brown & Co.
6. Jonsen AR, Siegler M & Winslade WJ. 1986. *Clinical Ethics*. MacMillan.
7. Tuckett D, Boulton M, Olson C & Williams A. 1985. *Meetings between Experts*. Tavistock Publications.
8. Waitzkin H. Nov 2 1874. Doctor–patient communication. *J Am Med Assoc.*, 17, 252.
9. Byrne FS & Long BEL. 1976. *Doctors Talking to Patients*. London: HMSO.
10. Pendleton D, Schofield T, Tate PHL & Havelock P. 1984. *The Consultation: An Approach to Learning and Teaching*. OUP.
11. Podell RN. 1975. *Physicians Guide to Compliance in Hypertension*. Merck.

12. King J, Pendleton D & Tate PHL. 1985. *Making the Most of Your Doctor*. Thames-Methuen.
13. RCGP. July 1985. 'What sort of doctor'. Report for General Practice No. 23.
14. Greenfield S, Kaplan S & Ware JE. 1985. Expanding patient involvement in care. *Ann Intern Med*. 102, 520–528.
15. Smith DH & Pettigrew LS. 1986. Mutual persuasion as a model for doctor–patient communication. *Theor Med*. 7 (2).
16. Katz J. 1984. *The Silent World of Doctor and Patient*. The Free Press (MacMillan).

CHAPTER 5

Joining the panel: All organisations are rife with cliques, rivalries, personal vendettas and greasy pole climbing. My father would have nothing to do with the RCGP, being certain it was populated by self-seeking, quasi-Masonic, pompous people with inferiority complexes. This was a widely held view then and is still current in some quarters even now. In his defence he did not like the BMA either. John Horder, one of my two trainers, had converted me and I had scraped through the 1974 examination. Not long after my joining the Panel I was taken to one side by a very senior member of Scottish extraction and told bluntly that he regretted my appointment, that I was yet another addition to the Oxford Mafia and that the College was in the grip of Oxford Mania, but I must tread carefully as this time was coming to an end. Bemused would not adequately describe my feelings. I had just been part of a very successful RCGP Spring Meeting in Oxford (1983), it had been very well received and a personal feather in the cap for John. It had not been received so well in some quarters apparently. He went on to point out that at that time, and it may be true still, the Council hated the (perceived) elitism of the bonded College examiners. They (Council thought) were too big for their boots and were an unelected, dangerous and anarchist tribe of superior intelligence. Truthfully, he didn't mention the last bit.

Fiona Godlee wrote an article just before John Foulkes arrived at the exam. At the time of writing, March 2020, she is editor of the BMJ.

Those of you who have the access can read the full article.

MRCGP: Examining the exam
Fiona Godlee: British Medical Journal, London WC I H 9J E Fiona Godlee, MRCP, assistant editor
BMJ 1991; 303:235-238, 27 JULY 1991

CHAPTER 6

Evidence for validity can come from a number of sources. Some involve the opinion of experts in the field; others require the collection of further data, to be used in an empirical validation; yet others involve the investigation of patterns of performance within a controlled setting or an examination. The notion of 'face' validity, meaning 'this looks sensible and relates to real issues' is widely used, but is often little more than a question of 'does this look OK?' Very important practical considerations, but purists would argue only on the periphery of what is meant by true validity.

Content validity is the extent to which the content of the instrument or assessment reflects the range of knowledge, skills or behaviours that are to be assessed, in the situations in which these are required. So that a first-year medical student could be assessed on their questioning and listening skills interviewing a 'normal' patient, while a final year student could be assessed breaking bad news or explaining treatment to patients and obtaining informed consent. The performance on a small number of similar items will be better correlated than performance on a larger number of different attributes. A doctor may be very good at explaining, but less effective in dealing with emotions and displaying empathy. There may therefore be a trade-off between the content validity of a measure and its internal consistency.

Another aspect of content validity might be the extent to which the evidence of competence which the assessor collects is representative of the generality of performance. This is a question both of sampling and of fidelity. The simulation may be a valid test of competence, but an inference of subsequent performance may be questionable, similarly a valid direct assessment of performance cannot be used to generalise about competence.

Criterion validity is the correlation between the item assessed and other measures of the same attribute. It is usually divided into two constructs, concurrent validity, comparing different methodologies measuring the same criterion, and predictive validity, in other words will the assessment of the consulting criteria predict subsequent outcomes?

Construct validity is acknowledged to be the most telling form of validity but the most difficult to establish. The question was how does the assessment relate to our hypotheses or constructs about what we were assessing? For example, if we are setting out to assess competent consulting, our assessment should be able to distinguish apprentices from masters. To a large extent, competence in consulting is acquired over time and is expected to bear a close relationship to experience for the majority of doctors; probably not a linear relationship, for there may come a point at which increasing experience implies declining competence. Again, if we are assessing the patient-centredness of a consultation, does our assessment correlate with measures of outcome for patients? Construct validity is established by a series of studies that can confirm the hypotheses and can be brought into question by a single study that refutes it. John made it clear that validity is a demanding concept that goes beyond asking a lot of people if they think you are doing the right thing.

We hid this paper away in an obscure American journal allowing quick publication to satisfy the requirements of the RCGP Exam Board.

Assessing Physicians' Interpersonal Skills via Videotaped Encounters: A New Approach for the Royal College of General Practitioners Membership Examination.*

The Royal College of General Practitioners' Membership examination, the only postgraduate qualification in family medicine in the United Kingdom, has developed a direct assessment of candidates' interpersonal skills performance using videotaped consultations of the actual doctor–patient encounters. At present about 1,200 doctors are examined each year. The methodology has been developed and piloted over a period of eight years. The central tenet of the methodology is a clear definition, which is known both to the candidate and to the examiner, of the clinical and consulting competencies that are required to be demonstrated in order to pass the examination. The candidate is required to provide evidence of his or her competence usually by selecting appropriate patient encounters that demonstrate the fulfillment of the required performance criteria, effectively producing a portfolio of his or her communicative competence. The methodology is intended to encourage the learning and teaching of communication skills by making it part of an important examination and clearly defining the competencies required to pass. Reliability has been demonstrated to be satisfactory and refinement of the marking processes is likely to improve this further.

Since its introduction in 1965, the examination for MRCGP has become one of the most respected and comprehensive primary care examinations in the world (Examining, 1990; Moore, 1998). Its validity and reliability are under constant review and as a consequence its format

* Tate P, Foulkes J, Neighbour R, Campion P, & Field S. 1999. Assessing physicians' interpersonal skills via videotaped encounters: A new approach for the Royal College of General Practitioners Membership examination. *J Health Commun.* 4(2), 143–152.

has changed over the years (Godlee, 1991). Until recently, however, it has not directly assessed the GP's clinical and interpersonal skills. This paper describes the development of a new instrument for assessing doctor–patient consulting skills, which has become part of the new modular MRCGP examination.

This was a necessary reform and followed the lead of the RCGP of Australia and New Zealand and the College of Family Physicians of Canada, which had already included clinical components in their examinations (Lockie, 1990; Wakeford, 1990). In 1990, the council of the RCGP instructed its examination board to devise a clinical component for the MRCGP. Videotape analysis of consultations was chosen because the technique had been widely used in medical and other health professional education for many years (Rutter & Maguire, 1976; Verby, 1976; Davis et al., 1980; Premi, 1991). It had proved to be relatively inexpensive, logistically feasible and familiar to most training practices (Martin & Martin, 1985; Field, 1995). The submitted videotape is also an enduring record of the candidate's performance, allowing scrutiny by several assessors at different times.

A video development group was formed, with a primary goal of developing a valid and reliable instrument to assess candidates' consultations. The secondary goal was that the assessment would also become an educational spur that would raise standards of consulting competence in general practice. The development group was always clear on the relationship between these two goals. If observed performance became part of the only UK postgraduate examination in general practice, then all potential candidates would need to consider aspects of their performance hitherto of low priority in relationship to examinations. The examination board intended the development to raise standards, particularly in establishing consulting competence as a subject worthy of assessment. There was a precedent for this aim. The introduction of the critical reading paper, an examination testing the candidate's knowledge of relevant literature and ability to critically read health-related academic papers, was implemented with another educational agenda to encourage candidates to read widely and critically. Research indicated that this objective was achieved (Lockie, 1990).

THE DEVELOPMENT OF PERFORMANCE CRITERIA

Some medical educators have tended to draw a distinction between competence and performance in which competence is considered to be a latent state of potentiality (i.e. what you know), whereas performance relates to the reality of day-to-day work (i.e. what you do; Rethans et al., 1990).

Video Assessment for Physician Certification

In assessment terms it is not altogether surprising that an assessment of competence thus defined, typically by means of indirect measures such as written examinations, may not relate very closely to actual performance. One of the major problems over recent decades has been both the feasibility of direct observation of large numbers of doctors and the criteria on which their performance should be judged (Rethans, Sturmans, Drop, van der Vleuten, & Hobus, 1990, 1991; Van der Vleuten, 1996). The development group sought to define competence in terms of the achievement of effective consultations in order both to take account of, and to possibly influence for the better, the outcome of the doctor–patient encounter.

The first step was to define the competencies required to satisfy the examiners. The development group agreed that the competencies should focus on the outcome of the doctor–patient encounters rather than specific styles of doctor behavior. There are many ways in which a doctor can arrive at the successful outcome of a consultation; there is no 'right' or 'wrong' way, although some ways are more effective than others. We did not wish to encourage particular styles of behaviour, running the risk of producing clones of doctors who all behaved in the same way. The wish was to encourage effective task-based consulting without being prescriptive on style. In order to achieve the clarity required some of the methodology of the National Vocational Qualification (NVQ) was adopted (Jessup, 1991). This is an examination method widely used in the United Kingdom and is essentially a workplace-orientated, task-centred descriptive assessment. The concept of task-based learning, teaching and assessment is well established in the medical literature (Pendleton, Schofield, Tate, & Havelock, 1984; Makoul, 1998), and a definition of clinical and consulting skill competence was derived from the relevant world literature (Balint, 1957; Byrne & Long, 1976; Stott & Davis, 1979; Tuckett, Boulton, Olson & Williams, 1985; Neighbour, 1987; Stewart, 1995).

The primary tasks of the family doctor were divided into five units:

- Discover the reasons for a patient's visit.
- Define the clinical problem(s).
- Explain the problem(s) to the patient.
- Address the patient's problem(s).
- Make effective use of the consultation.

Each of these units was subdivided into elements. For example, in unit one, 'Discover the reasons for a patient's visit', there were four elements:

- Elicit the patient's account of the symptom(s) that made him or her turn to the doctor.
- Obtain relevant items of social and occupational circumstances.
- Explore the patient's health understanding.
- Inquire about continuing problems.

Even at the element level it was felt that these tasks were too broad to be reliably assessed. Therefore, more specific performance criteria (PCs) were defined. Each element of the definition has one or more PCs. The units and elements were derived by an assimilation of the literature relating to clinical and consulting competence as appropriate to British general practice. The PCs were derived by interviewing the members of the working party who were practising GPs, encouraging them to dissect out the performance tasks required to achieve the higher level elements and units. The question asked was, 'What must happen for that to be achieved?' Thus, for the unit, 'Discover the reasons for a patient's visit' and the element 'Elicit the patient's account of the symptom(s) that made him or her turn to the doctor', there are two PCs:

- The doctor encourages the patient's contribution at appropriate points in the consultation.
- The doctor responds to cues.

At this time the full definition of doctor–patient communication competence included the five units along with 16 elements and 21 PCs. The original intention of the working party was that this definition in its entirety would form the basis of the assessment of candidates and that the judgements would be made at the level of the PCs. During the initial piloting phase from 1991 to 1994 a major flaw in this strategy became apparent. The doctors being assessed were typically just at the end of their vocational training course for family medicine, a three-year course with two years in a hospital and one year in supervised practice. They are mostly in their late 20s. When these young doctors' performances were scrutinized using the full definition, an unacceptably high level of failure was found of up to 80%. Was the definition simply too encompassing and unrealistic? To test this question, we asked some examiners and their established partners, a total of 40 experienced GPs, to submit videotaped encounters to be assessed. Even when applying the full definition, they all passed, most very easily.

In order to fashion the tool to realistically assess young doctors just at the end of vocational training, the Panel of Examiners was consulted using a modified 'Delphi' technique. The Panel, 130 strong at this time and all practising GPs from the United Kingdom and Eire, was given the full definition of competence and asked to rate which performance criteria should be mandatory in order to pass the MRCGP examination. If over 50% of the Panel agreed the PC was deemed mandatory, using this methodology seven PCs were made mandatory. Perhaps unsurprisingly these initial criteria were very 'doctor centered' (Byrne & Long, 1976). Further piloting suggested the criteria were perhaps too basic and were really working at the level of minimal competence rather than the optimal competence level expected by the RCGP examination board. So, two years after the first Delphi consultation, the Panel of Examiners was consulted again. This produced an additional four PCs, making 11 in all (Table A.1).

A concern of the development group was the problem of assessing both clinical and consulting skills in the one examination. The evidence for the 'generalisability' of a doctor's consulting skills seemed initially to be compelling (Byrne & Long, 1976; Tuckett, Boulton, Olson, & Williams, 1985), while it was also clear that a doctor's clinical performance was likely to be more case specific. Nevertheless, to observe the reality of a GP's performance in the workplace, the two sets of skills, clinical and communication, intertwine. Within the blueprint of the examination it is clear that the video

Table A.1 The Mandatory Performance Criteria to be Demonstrated for Examinations in 1996 and 1997

1. The doctor encourages the patient's contribution at appropriate points in the consultation.
2. The doctor responds to cues.
3. The doctor elicits appropriate details to place the complaint(s) in a social and psychological context.
4. The doctor obtains sufficient information for no serious condition to be missed.
5. The doctor chooses an examination which is likely to confirm or disprove hypotheses which could reasonably have been formed OR is designed to address a patient's concern.
6. The doctor appears to make a clinically appropriate working diagnosis.
7. The doctor explains the diagnosis, management and effects of treatment.
8. The doctor explains in language appropriate to the patient.
9. The doctor's management plan is appropriate for the working diagnosis, reflecting a good understanding of modern accepted medical practice.
10. The doctor shares management options with the patient.
11. The doctor's prescribing behaviour is appropriate.

assessment is a good test of verbal and non-verbal communication. It also assesses 'real life' clinical problem solving, patient management, some values and attitudes, and (by means of the workbook, which will be described later) self-appraisal skills. Other parts of the exam assess clinical ability.

To be an effective educational tool the methodology had to allow constructive feedback to the candidate in the event of a failure within this component of the examination. This is in the spirit of the examination being an integral part of the educational process. The use of specific performance criteria allows this; candidates can be informed about which performance criteria they failed to provide evidence of competence. This explicit information should enable such candidates to concentrate on areas of performance highlighted by the assessment and to resubmit further evidence with increased confidence.

THE ASSESSMENT PROCESS

Candidates are currently required to submit a VHS videotape containing 15 consultations in order to allow a sufficient case mix given the varied nature of general practice consultations and the problem of patient refusal. Candidates are asked to include at least two consultations with children under 10 years of age and at least two consultations involving chronic disease in adult patients. They are recommended to mainly include consultations for new problems, as they are more likely to demonstrate a wider range of the criteria than with uncomplicated follow-up appointments. Because these young doctors are mostly in training posts, many of the patients are new to them.

The candidates complete a workbook to accompany their videotape. The workbook was developed to alert assessors of the context and nature of the consultations. It has become a useful educational tool in its own right. It consists of a log of all consultations with timings, 15 consultation assessment forms and five minute-by-minute consultation description forms. Candidates are asked to select five consultations that most demonstrate their competence and to complete the description forms for these.

In addition, the workbook contains detailed instructions, including the full definition of competence with the mandatory PCs clearly marked. Advice on recording, patient consent forms and extracts from the RCGP ethical guidelines are also included. Our approach to the assessment of competence is therefore that the candidate:

- Knows the competencies that must be demonstrated.
- Conforms to rules governing the submission of evidence.
- Is guided by a mentor or trainer.
- Submits evidence when it is ready.

From the candidate's point of view, the assessors wish them to submit a videotape with a range of challenge that clearly demonstrates their current consulting ability. The tape can be looked on as a portfolio of competence.

EVALUATION OF THE VIDEO ASSESSMENT

The utility of an assessment method can be evaluated by considering five qualities: reliability, validity, feasibility, acceptability and educational impact. It is the balance and the mix that is important to the success of any assessment tool.

Reliability

In November 1997, during the third operational assessment of the MRCGP tapes, an exercise was undertaken to investigate the extent of inter-rater reliability. Tapes were assessed initially by one pair of examiners watching seven consultations. Where competence had not been established, the tape was passed to a second pair, who also watched seven consultations, six of which were previously not seen, so that up to 13 would be examined. This second pair made a pass/fail decision. One hundred tapes were used in the reliability study: all 58 tapes that were failed and a randomised selection of 42 tapes drawn from the 341 passing tapes, which were returned and submitted to the full process as described above. Only the final outcome of the whole process was used as input to the data set. For example, a tape that was passed only after being seen by a second pair of examiners during the routine assessment, but that was passed by the first pair in the research assessment, was considered to have passed in both instances. This is because the assessors in the research exercise had no knowledge of which consultations had been seen previously, and the first pair of research assessors was most unlikely to make the same selection of consultations as the first pair of routine assessors.

Table A.2 Reliability exercise results[a]

| Second viewing | | | |
First viewing	Fail	Pass	Total
Fail	47	11	58
Pass	0	42	42
Total	47	53	100

[a] The agreement between the first and the second viewing was measured by the phi coefficient (0.80) and by Cohen's kappa (0.78).

The second pair of examiners also passed all 42 passing tapes. Of the 58 failing tapes, the second pair also failed 47 and 11 were passed. See Table A.2.

The level of agreement was encouraging, given that this was the third operational marking session using assessors who, for the most part, are quite familiar with the method. Support is now being given to assessors through plenary discussions and through the monitoring and evaluation of smaller groups of assessors in a rolling programme. Piloting is continuing in order to refine the methodology and improve the reliability even further.

In this assessment of consulting skills, examiner judgement is central. The examiners are guided by performance criteria (which are also available to the candidate) and their internalised notion of the acceptable standard is shared, as far as possible, by working together – in pairs, in small groups and in plenary sessions. However, it remains true that the pass/fail line falls at the point of maximum uncertainty between the poles of obvious success and obvious failure. Given this, it is surprising that there were no tapes that were passed in the routine assessment and failed in the research exercise. There is overall a preponderance of passing tapes (approximately 85% in this study) and possibly a predisposition on the part of examiners to pass marginal candidates rather than to fail them. Development of the marking methodology to allow more examiners to see the consultations of one candidate are being piloted in order to minimise this bias.

Validity

The PCs were produced with reference to a wide literature search and then were modified by consultation with over 100 practising GPs. Because of this approach, the instrument appears to have good content validity. They are all associated with process outcomes such as patient compliance or satisfaction and are widely accepted throughout the profession (Stewart, 1995). The PCs are also all contained in the recent GMC guidance describing good medical practice (General Medical Council, 1995). That document was developed separately and therefore provides powerful corroboration.

Feasibility and Acceptability

The feasibility has now been tested on a national scale and found to be workable and no more onerous or expensive than the MRCGP oral examinations. There have been some concerns about the increasing workload of MRCGP examiners, but changes in the examining environment (making it residential and moving to group marking of a single candidate while retaining the two-stage process described above) has improved the acceptability of the process. It may soon be possible to regionalise the marking to make it easier for examiners. Many candidates have found the preparation onerous and time consuming. The working party has redesigned and simplified the workbook and reduced the number of consultations required from 24 to 15, with a further reduction in prospect, to address some of these concerns. Patient acceptance has for the most part been excellent; almost all candidates reported little or no difficulty. For a few, however, there was considerable frustration when they were denied permission to record their more effective consultations by the patients, but this is apparently an infrequent event (Coleman & Manku-Scott, 1998).

Educational Impact and the Future Development of the MRCGP Video Assessment Instrument

In 1998 the MRCGP examination adopted a modular format. The videotaped consulting skills assessment is one of the four new modules. The requirements of the reorganised examination means that the video assessment has to be able to award a 'merit' pass as well as making a just pass/fail decision. To achieve this end, all 100 trained video examiners took part in a third modified 'Delphi' exercise to ascertain if there were any PCs that should become mandatory and what PCs should be demonstrated in order to be awarded a merit. This process has resulted in the addition of one further mandatory PC and three new 'merit' PCs. The merit criteria are as follows:

1. *Unit*: Discover the reasons for a patient's visit.
   Element: Explore the patient's health understanding.
   PC: The doctor takes the patient's health understanding into account.

2. *Unit*: Explain the problem(s) to the patient.
   Element: Tailor the explanation to the patient.
   PC: The doctor explains to the patient utilising some or all of the patient's elicited beliefs.

3. *Unit*: Explain the problem(s) to the patient.
   Element: Ensure that the explanation is understood and accepted by the patient.
   PC: The doctor tries to confirm the patient's understanding.

The video development group hopes that the selection of these obviously patient-centred criteria will send a clear message to candidates and the educational establishment as to the type of doctor–patient consulting the RCGP wishes to encourage. We hope shortly to be able to report on the pattern of patient-centred behaviour in candidates who submit themselves for the examination.

Examiner training will continue to be developed, as will strict quality control measures. Material for candidates, including books (Moore, 1998; Tate, 1997) and videotapes (Skelton, Field, Tate, & Wiskin, 1998), are growing in number. In the light of the experience of the first two examinations, attempts have been made to lessen the burden on candidates. For instance, consultations should not be longer than 15 minutes and the 'mapping' exercise has been discarded in favour of a modified self-evaluation proforma.

Summary

A method has been devised for assessing the professional competence of GPs using direct observation of actual performance in the usual place of work via videotape recording. A coherent approach to the assessment of competence provides a rationale for the selection of evidence, which must be outside the control of the examiners. In fact, this assessment implies a transfer of control from examiner to candidate. The candidate knows what must be demonstrated and is given ample opportunity to gather the evidence, effectively being asked to produce a portfolio of competence.

The method is transparently a criterion-referenced form of assessment. Professional competence is predefined using the unit, element and PC structure used in NVQs. Competence is judged to be either present or absent. The Panel of Examiners sets the standard before any candidate is assessed and is not determined by arbitrary post hoc inspection of scores. There is an expectation that most candidates will be successful, but those who fail are given exact reasons for the failure, fulfilling the educational rationale behind the development. The method allows for the introduction of further performance criteria both at pass and merit level in order to encourage and keep pace with the expected improvement in consulting competence. The instrument has been demonstrated to have acceptable reliability and is likely to influence the development of consulting behaviour in UK GPs to the benefit of their patients.

References

1. Balint M. 1957. *The Doctor, His Patient and the Illness*. Edinburgh: Churchill Livingston.
2. Byrne P & Long B. 1976. *Doctors Talking to Patients*. London: Royal College of General Practitioners Publications.
3. Coleman T & Manku-Scott T. 1998. Comparison of video-recorded consultations with those in which patients' consent is withheld. *BJGP*. 48, 971–974.
4. Cronbach LJ. 1951. Coefficient alpha and the internal structure of tests. *Psychometrika*. 16, 297–334.
5. Cronbach LJ, Gleser GC, Nanda H & Rajaratnam N. *The Dependability of Behavioural Measurements: Theory of Generalizability for Scores and Profiles*. New York: Wiley, 1972.

6. Davis RH, Jenkins M, Smail SA, Stott NCH, Verby JE & Wallace BB. 1980. Teaching with audio-visual recordings of consultations. *J R Coll Gen Pract.* 30, 333–336.

7. Field S. 1995. The use of video recording in general practice education: A survey of trainers in the West Midlands region. *Educ Gen Pract.* 6, 49–58.

8. General Medical Council. 1995. *Good Medical Practice.* London: General Medical Council.

9. Godlee F. 1990. Examining the Royal Colleges examinations [Editorial]. *Lancet*, 335, 443.

10. Godlee F. 1991. MRCGP. Examining the exam. *BMJ.* 303, 235–238.

11. Jessup G. 1991. *Outcomes: NVQs and the Emerging Model of Education and Training.* London: Falmer Press.

12. Lockie C. (Ed.). 1990. *The Examination for Membership of the Royal College of General Practitioners (MRCGP): Development, Current State and Future Trends. Occasional Paper 46.* London: Royal College of General Practitioners.

13. Makoul G. 1998. Communication research in medical education. In: LD Jackson & BK Duffy (Eds.), *Health Communication Research: A Guide to Developments and Directions.* Westport, CT: Greenwood Publishing Group.

14. Martin E & Martin PM. 1985. The reactions of patients to a video camera in the consulting room. *J R Coll Gen Pract.* 34, 607–610.

15. Moore R. 1998. *The MRCGP Examination: A Guide for Candidates and Teachers*, 3rd ed. London: Royal College of General Practitioners.

16. Neighbour R. 1987. *The Inner Consultation.* London: Kluwer Academic Publishers.

17. Pendleton D, Schofield T, Tate P & Havelock P. 1984. *The Consultation: An Approach to Learning and Teaching.* Oxford: Oxford University Press.

18. Premi J. 1991. An assessment of 15 years' experience in using videotape review in a family practice residency. *Acad Med.* 66, 56–57.

19. Rethans JJ, Sturmans F, Drop R., van der Vleuten C & Hobus P. 1990. Competence and performance: Two different concepts in the assessment of quality of medical care. *Fam Pract.* 7, 168–174.

20. Rethans JJ, Sturmans F, Drop R, van der Vleuten C & Hobus P. 1991. Does competence of general practitioners predict their performance? Comparison between examination setting and actual practice. *BMJ.* 303, 1377–1380.

21. Rutter DR & Maguire GP. 1976. History-taking for medical students: Evaluation of a training programme. *Lancet.* ii, 558–560.

22. Skelton J, Field S, Tate P, & Wiskin C. (Eds.). 1998. *Those Things You Say [Videotape]*. Oxford: Radcliffe Medical Press.
23. Stewart M. 1995. Effective physician-patient communication and health outcomes: A review. *Can Med Assoc J.* 45, 137–141.
24. Stott N & Davis R. 1979. The exceptional potential in each primary care consultation. *J. R Coll Gen Pract.* 29, 201–205.
25. Streiner N & Norman GR. *Health Measurement Scales: A Practical Guide to Their Development and Use*, 2nd ed. Oxford: Oxford University Press, 1995.
26. Tate P. 1997. *The Doctor's Communication Handbook*, 2nd ed. Oxford: Radcliffe Medical Press.
27. Tuckett D, Boulton M, Olson C & Williams A. 1985. *Meetings between Experts*. London: Tavistock Publications.
28. Van der Vleuten C. 1996. The assessment of professional competence: Developments, research and practical implications. *Adv Health Sci Educ.* 1, 41–67.
29. Verby JE. 1976. The audio-visual interview. A new tool in medical education. *JAMA.* 236, 2413–2414.
30. Wakeford R. 1990. International background. In: C Lockie (Ed.), *The Examination for the Membership of the Royal College of General Practitioners (MRCGP): Development, Current State and Future Trends. Occasional Paper 46*. London: Royal College of General Practitioners.

This is the discussion section of the paper Peter Campion produced in 2002.

Patient centredness in the MRCGP video examination: Analysis of large cohort

(Published 28 September 2002) BMJ 2002;325:691

'These results show that effective, patient-centred, consulting as currently defined by the MRCGP exam is uncommon. Candidates have no difficulty demonstrating their competence in traditional 'medical' skills of asking questions, choosing appropriate physical examinations, making diagnoses, prescribing, explaining and achieving rapport. However, when tested against operationalised criteria for patient-centredness, which are on the face of it not difficult things to do (asking patients for their views of their illness, how their life is affected or how they feel about their illness, and asking simply whether they understand

what has been said), very few candidates actually do this in more than one or two of their submitted consultations.

No assessment is perfect but represents a compromise between rigour and feasibility. Some candidates may have difficulty recording themselves and those who take more time and record more sessions are more likely to succeed. The assessors have noticed however remarkable consistencies of behaviour despite these provisos. Videotape assessment still stands at the top of Miller's Pyramid:

Does
Shows how
Knows how
Knows.

Simulation as in the simulated surgery option is at the 'shows how' level, the oral examination examines 'knows how' and written examinations are at the 'knows' level.

There has been much debate in the last decade about how measurements of competence predict performance in real life. These results demonstrate that only direct observation reveals what doctors actually do in the consulting room. Inferences about performance drawn from other test modalities, such as written or oral examinations, are likely to be inaccurate.

We have found that effective patient-centred consulting is an unusual behaviour in MRCGP candidates: based on all the criteria, only about one in ten candidates demonstrated such behaviour on a regular basis. This confirms the recent findings of Stevenson et al. of the rarity of shared decision making. Effective checking of patients' understanding is even rarer. We have to conclude that the core of the discipline of general practice – being able to communicate effectively with patients – is not easy to achieve. Most doctors at the end of a long period of training seem not to have mastered these skills, despite professing belief in their importance. (We can only speculate at the extent of patient-centredness among junior hospital doctors.) It may be that there is a 'time and experience' factor involved, and that patient-centredness increases over the years. Indeed, our initial pilots during development of the method, using tapes supplied by examiners and their partners, suggest that this might well be the case. Recent work by Howie et al. suggests that 'patient enablement' is more likely when the GP knows the patient well, though this is not an essential proviso. We have demonstrated that the majority of candidates for the MRCGP examination have not yet acquired a participative (enabling) style of communication. However, we are convinced of the evidence that, with the information explosion and an increasing expectation for patients to be more involved in their own care, doctors need to be able to consult in patient-centred ways. Instilling this ability more reliably into doctors of whatever age and experience is a major challenge to the vocational training establishment, to medical educationalists and to those hoping to ensure that revalidation will bring benefits to the care of patients'.

Here are some graphed incidences of observed consulting behaviour from the 2000/2001 cohort (~14,000 consultations).

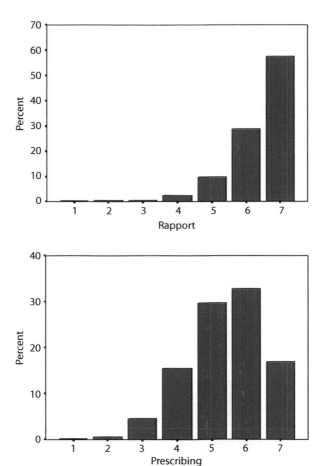

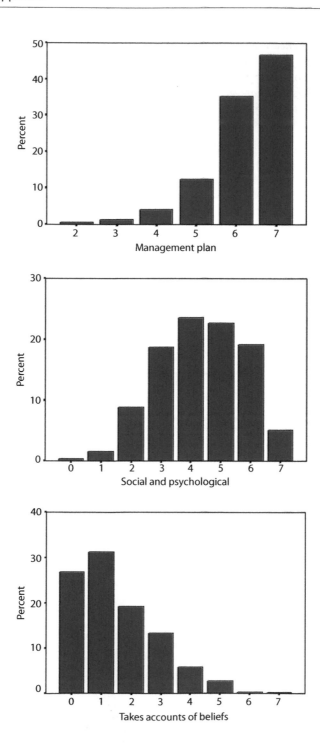

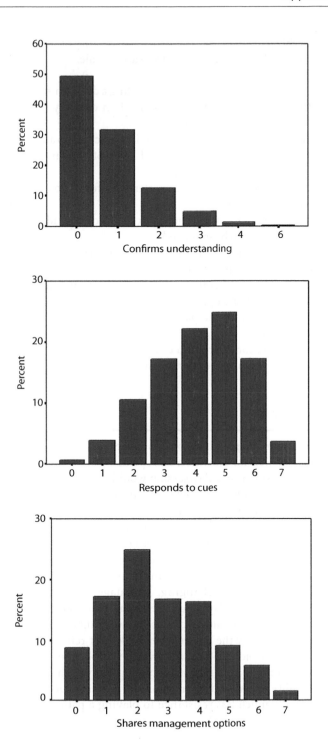

In 2006 this paper further established the validity of the methodology. Using a previously validated OPTIONS rating scale.

- The clinician identifies a problem(s) needing a decision-making process.
- The clinician states that there is more than one way to deal with an identified problem ('equipoise').
- The clinician lists 'options', including the choice of 'no action' if feasible.
- The clinician explains the pros and cons of options to the patient (taking 'no action' is an option).
- The clinician checks the patient's preferred information format (words/numbers/visual display).
- The clinician explores the patient's expectations (or ideas) about how the problem(s) are to be managed.
- The clinician explores the patient's concerns (fears) about how problem(s) are to be managed.
- The clinician checks that the patient has understood the information.
- The clinician provides opportunities for the patient to ask questions.
- The clinician asks for the patient's preferred level of involvement in decision making.
- An opportunity for deferring a decision is provided.
- Arrangements are made to review the decision (or the deferment).

CHAPTER 7

Twenty-five years of running courses honed a technique that worked internationally well for Northern Europeans, Russians, Americans, UK and Eire. The first part of a day/session would be based on the task-based theories of the consultation, cycles of care and discussion. The second part was much more bespoke and prone to modification on the hoof. The underlying aim was to get the medical participants to really feel what it was like to be a patient, so the central tool was role-play, or on some occasions using actors. In some ways the role-play was better as that person really did find themselves in the patients mind and these insights were often revelatory and behaviour changing. Language was only important in the debriefing, the role-plays could be in the group's language, Russian, Icelandic, whatever. The rules of discussion were highlighted, though over the years I used to give the 'patient' feedback freer rein.

Most doctors avoid role-play, for a variety of obvious reasons, but it is the role of doctor they are afraid of, surprising really as I have always felt the very artificiality was a good defence for self-perceived poor performance. There is usually much less resistance to playing a patient and this is the experience most likely to help them. I used to prepare several scripts that were linked to contemporary research so that when the discussion phase arrived there was clear evidence to confirm or refute the opinions being offered. This evidence changed over time, but the structure did not. This was before smartphones and widespread Google, but some prior research is still a must. Here are a few examples:

As a warm-up exercise: What is it like on the other side of the fence? Groups of three to four, two to three minutes each. One member be prepared to summarise briefly the salient points.

Think of the last time you were ill enough to go to a doctor. Why did you go? What were you hoping for? Did you get what you wanted? What was good? What could have been improved?

And now the evidence, usually on PowerPoint slides to be used only if appropriate.

Index

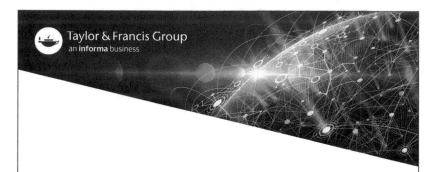